A

COMPLETE MANUAL

ON HEALTH

AND

VITALITY

BY

KELVIN WILLIAMS

Copyright © 2023 Kelvin Williams

All rights reserved

ISBN: 9798857464663

You can reach me through my author center page by scanning the bar code bellow

DEDICATION

This book is dedicated to my late parents Mr. and Mrs. Williams.

TABLE OF CONTENT

ACKNOWLEDGMENTS

I am deeply grateful to everyone who supported me in bringing this book to life, "A Comparative Guide to Wellness and Vitality." Writing this book has been a journey of passion and dedication, and I couldn't have accomplished it without the help and encouragement of numerous individuals.

First and foremost, I want to thank my family sincerely for their constant support during this project. Your love, patience, and understanding provided the foundation upon which I built this book.

I extend my heartfelt appreciation to my friends and colleagues who offered valuable insights and feedback during the research and writing process. Your discussions and perspectives enriched the content and helped shape the final product.

I am indebted to the experts and practitioners in the fields of wellness and vitality who generously shared their knowledge and experiences. Your contributions have added depth and credibility to the information presented in this guide.

Last but not least, I want to express my appreciation to my readers. Your interest in exploring the realms of wellness and vitality is what drives authors like me to continue creating meaningful content.

We appreciate your participation in this adventure. Your support has been a constant source of inspiration, and I am honored to share this book with you.

Sincerely,

[Kelvin Williams]

CHAPTER ONE

WELLNESS AND VITALITY

Wellness and vitality are essential aspects of leading a healthy and fulfilling life. In today's fast-paced world, where various factors can contribute to stress, sedentary lifestyles, and poor dietary choices, understanding and prioritizing wellness and vitality have become increasingly important.

Wellness refers to a state of holistic well-being that encompasses various dimensions of health, including physical, mental, emotional, social, and spiritual well-being. It's not just the absence of illness but also the presence of positive factors that contribute to a high quality of life. Achieving wellness involves making conscious choices and adopting behaviors that promote overall health.

Vitality, on the other hand, specifically emphasizes a sense of energy, vibrancy, and enthusiasm for life. It's about feeling alive, active, and engaged in daily activities. Vitality is closely linked to physical health, mental clarity, and emotional balance. When you have vitality, you're not just going through the motions but embracing life with zest.

Here are some key components and tips related to wellness and vitality:

1. Physical Wellness:

- Regular exercise: Take part in physical pursuits you enjoy, such dancing, yoga, or jogging.

- Balanced nutrition: Consume a variety of nutrient-rich foods, including fruits, vegetables, whole grains, lean proteins, and healthy fats.

- Enough sleep: Make 7-9 hours of good sleep a priority each night.

- Regular check-ups: Visit healthcare professionals for routine check-ups and screenings.

2. Mental Wellness:

- Stress management: Practice relaxation techniques like deep breathing, meditation, or mindfulness to manage stress.

- Cognitive stimulation: Keep your mind active by reading, learning new skills, or solving puzzles.

- Positive mindset: Cultivate optimism and practice self-compassion to foster mental well-being.

3. Emotional Wellness:

- Express emotions: Allow yourself to feel and express your emotions in a healthy way.

- Social connections: Build and maintain supportive

relationships with friends and family.

- Seek help: If needed, don't hesitate to reach out to mental health professionals for guidance.

4. Social Wellness:

- Connect with others: Engage in social activities, join clubs, or participate in community events.

- Communication skills: Develop effective communication skills to build and nurture relationships.

5. Spiritual Wellness:

- Reflect and meditate: Spend time in self-reflection and meditation to connect with your inner self.

- Take part in worthwhile activities: Take part in pursuits that are consistent with your ideals and give you a sense of direction.

6. Lifestyle Choices:

- Avoid harmful habits: Limit or avoid substances like alcohol, tobacco, and recreational drugs.

- Work-life balance: Strive for a healthy balance between work, leisure, and personal time.

Remember that wellness and vitality are interconnected. When you prioritize one aspect, it often positively impacts others. It's an ongoing journey that requires conscious effort, self-awareness, and the willingness to make positive changes. By nurturing your overall well-being, you can enhance your vitality and lead a more fulfilling life.

Prioritizing vitality, which refers to the state of being strong, active, and energetic, is crucial for various aspects of our well-being and overall quality of life. Here are some reasons highlighting the importance of prioritizing vitality:

1. Physical Health: Vitality is closely tied to physical health. When you prioritize vitality, you are more likely to engage in regular exercise, maintain a balanced diet, and get enough sleep. These factors contribute to a strong immune system, a healthy weight, and a reduced risk of chronic diseases like diabetes, heart disease, and certain cancers.

2. Mental Well-being: Physical vitality has a significant impact on mental well-being. Regular exercise is known to release endorphins; the "feel-good" hormones that can help lessen stress, anxiety, and sadness. When you feel physically vital, it can lead to improved self-esteem and a positive self-image.

3. Energy and Productivity: Vitality provides you with the energy and stamina necessary to be productive in your daily activities. Whether it's excelling in your professional life, participating in hobbies, or engaging in social interactions, having ample energy allows you

to do more and feel accomplished.

4. Cognitive Function: Exercise and a healthy lifestyle have been linked to improved cognitive function and brain health. Prioritizing vitality can enhance your focus, memory, and overall cognitive abilities, helping you stay sharp and mentally agile as you age.

5. Quality of Life: Feeling vital and energetic enhances your overall quality of life. You can actively participate in activities you enjoy, travel, explore new interests, and engage in meaningful relationships. This leads to a more fulfilling and satisfying life.

6. Longevity: Research suggests that maintaining a healthy lifestyle and prioritizing vitality can contribute to increased lifespan. By reducing the risk of chronic illnesses and maintaining physical and mental well-being, you are more likely to live a longer, healthier life.

7. Positive Influence: When you prioritize vitality, you set a positive example for those around you, such as family, friends, and colleagues. Your commitment to a healthy lifestyle can inspire others to make positive changes in their own lives.

8. Stress Management: A strong sense of vitality can help you better cope with stress. Engaging in physical activity, practicing relaxation techniques, and taking care of your body can improve your resilience and ability to handle life's challenges.

9. Preventive Care: Prioritizing vitality involves taking proactive steps to prevent health issues rather than just reacting to them. Regular exercise, a balanced diet, and other healthy habits can serve as effective preventive measures against various health conditions.

10. Happiness and Well-being: Vitality is closely linked to happiness and well-being. When you feel vital and healthy, you're more likely to experience a positive outlook on life and a greater sense of overall happiness.

In essence, prioritizing vitality is not just about looking good; it's about feeling good, both physically and mentally. By making conscious choices to take care of your body and mind, you can experience numerous benefits that positively impact various aspects of your life.

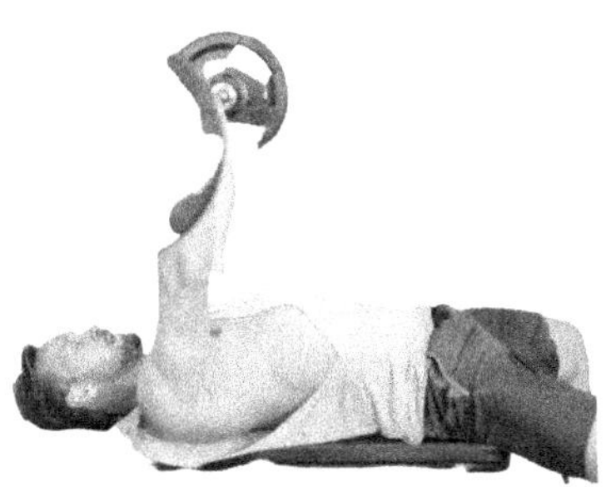

CHAPTER TWO

NUTRITION AND BALANCED DIET

Nutrition and a balanced diet are essential for maintaining good health and well-being. A balanced diet provides the necessary nutrients, energy, and other components that the body needs to function optimally. Here's an overview of the key aspects of nutrition and a balanced diet:

1. Nutrients:

Nutrients are substances that the body needs for growth, development, and overall functioning. Nutrients fall into six primary categories:

Carbohydrates: Provide energy.

- Proteins: Essential for tissue repair, growth, and immune function.

- Fats: Vital for storing energy, providing insulation, and safeguarding organs.

- Vitamins: Support various biochemical processes in the body.

- Minerals: Essential for bone health, nerve function, and more.

- Water: Vital for hydration, temperature regulation, and biochemical reactions.

2. Balanced Diet:

A balanced diet involves consuming the right amounts of nutrients from various food groups to ensure optimal health. The key food groups include:

- Fruits and vegetables: Packed with nutrients like fiber, antioxidants, vitamins, and minerals.

- Grains: Provide carbohydrates, fiber, and some essential nutrients.

- Lean meats, poultry, fish, beans, legumes, nuts, and seeds are good sources of protein.

- Dairy or Dairy Alternatives: Important sources of calcium and vitamin D.

- Fats and Oils: Choose healthy fats like those found in avocados, nuts, and olive oil.

3. Importance of Balance:

A balanced diet helps prevent deficiencies and chronic diseases such as obesity, heart disease, diabetes, and certain cancers. Each nutrient plays a unique role, so it's important not to overemphasize one nutrient at the expense of others.

4. Portion Control:

Eating the right portion sizes is crucial. Even eating nutritious meals in excess can result in weight gain. Pay attention to portion sizes to prevent consuming too many calories. Intake

5. Nutritional Recommendations:

The specific nutritional needs vary based on factors such as age, sex, physical activity level, and health status. Nutritional guidelines such as the Dietary Guidelines for Americans or similar guidelines in other countries provide recommendations for various age groups and dietary preferences.

6. Hydration:

Digestion, circulation, and temperature control are just a few of the body processes that water is crucial for. Keep yourself hydrated by consuming enough water throughout the day.

7. Moderation and Variety:

Enjoy a variety of foods to ensure you get a wide range of nutrients. Moderation is key, even with healthy foods. Avoid excessive consumption of sugary, high-fat, and processed foods.

8. Individualization:

Nutrition needs can differ widely among individuals. Consulting a registered dietitian or healthcare professional can provide personalized guidance based on your specific requirements and goals.

Incorporating these principles into your daily eating habits can contribute to better health and overall well-being. Remember that consistency over time is more important than occasional deviations, and it's okay to enjoy treats in moderation while primarily focusing on nutrient-dense foods.

Macronutrients and micronutrients

are essential components of our diet that provide the necessary energy and support for various bodily functions. They are necessary to preserve general health and wellbeing. Let's delve into each of them:

Macronutrients:

Macronutrients are nutrients that are required by the body in relatively large amounts to provide energy and support various physiological functions. The following three categories of macronutrients dominate:

1. Carbohydrates: The body's main fuel source is carbohydrates.

They are broken down into glucose, which is used by cells for energy. Foods rich in carbohydrates include grains (bread, rice, and pasta), fruits, vegetables, and legumes.

2. Proteins: Proteins are crucial for building and repairing tissues, supporting immune function, and

serving as enzymes and hormones. They are composed of amino acids, which are the building blocks of the body. Meat, poultry, fish, eggs, dairy products, legumes, nuts, and seeds are all excellent sources of protein.

3. Fats: Fats are another energy source and are essential for absorbing fat-soluble vitamins (A, D, E, and K). They also play a role in cell structure and provide insulation for the body. Healthy fat sources include avocados, nuts, seeds, olive oil, and fatty fish.

Micronutrients:

Micronutrients are nutrients required by the body in smaller amounts but are equally important for maintaining good health. They don't provide energy directly but are essential for various physiological processes. Micronutrients include vitamins and minerals:

1. Vitamins: Vitamins are organic compounds that are necessary for various bodily functions. They often act as coenzymes or cofactors, assisting enzymes in their functions. Vitamins are classified into water-soluble (e.g., vitamin C, B vitamins) and fat-soluble (e.g., vitamins A, D, E, and K). They play roles in immune function, bone health, vision, skin health, and more.

2. Minerals: Minerals are inorganic elements that play important roles in various bodily functions, including bone health, nerve transmission, fluid balance, and

enzyme activity. Calcium, iron, magnesium, potassium, and zinc are a few minerals.

It's important to maintain a balanced diet that includes adequate amounts of both macronutrients and micronutrients. Consuming a variety of foods from different food groups can help ensure you're getting the right balance of these essential nutrients for optimal health and well-being. If you have specific dietary concerns or goals, consulting a registered dietitian or healthcare professional is recommended.

Meal planning and portion control are essential aspects of maintaining a healthy and balanced diet. They can help you achieve your nutritional goals, manage your weight, and ensure you're getting the right nutrients in the right amounts. Here's a guide on how to effectively approach meal planning and portion control:

Meal Planning:

1. Set Your Goals: Determine what you want to achieve with your diet. Whether its weight loss, muscle gain, improved energy levels, or better overall health, your goals will shape your meal plan.

2. Choose Nutrient-Dense Foods: Focus on whole, minimally processed foods that are rich in nutrients. Include a variety of fruits, vegetables, lean proteins, whole grains, and healthy fats in your plan.

3. Plan Your Meals: Create a weekly meal plan that includes breakfast, lunch, dinner, and snacks. This prevents last-minute unhealthy choices and helps you stay on track.

4. Consider Caloric Needs: Calculate your daily caloric needs based on your goals and activity level. Make sure your meals align with these caloric requirements.

5. Prep in Advance: Prepare some meals and ingredients in advance to save time during busy days. Prepping ingredients can also make it easier to assemble meals quickly.

6. Include Snacks: Plan for healthy snacks to prevent excessive hunger between meals. Opt for options like nuts, yogurt, fruits, and veggies with hummus.

7. Variety is Key: Aim for a variety of foods to ensure you're getting a wide range of nutrients. Different colors, textures, and flavors in your meals can also make eating more enjoyable.

Portion Control:

1. Use Portion Control Tools: Familiarize yourself with portion control tools, such as measuring cups, a kitchen scale, and visual cues. This helps you understand what a proper portion looks like.

2. Read Labels: Pay attention to serving sizes on food labels. They can be quite different from what you might consider a portion.

3. Listen to Your Body: Eat slowly and pay attention to your body's hunger and fullness cues. When you are comfortably full but not overstuffed, stop eating.

4. Plate Composition: Use the "plate method" as a guide: Fill half your plate with non-starchy vegetables, a quarter with lean protein, and a quarter with whole grains or starchy vegetables.

5. Avoid Eating from Packages: Portion out snacks and meals onto a plate or bowl instead of eating directly from a package. This prevents mindless overeating.

6. Stay Mindful: Avoid distractions while eating, such as watching TV or using your phone. Being present during meals can help you recognize when you're full.

7. Small Changes: Gradually reduce portion sizes if you're used to larger portions. Your stomach will adjust over time.

Remember, meal planning and portion control are about finding a sustainable and enjoyable way of eating. It's not about strict deprivation or rigid rules. It's essential to create a plan that fits your lifestyle and preferences while still promoting your health and wellness goals. If you're unsure about your dietary needs or have specific health concerns, consider consulting a registered dietitian or nutritionist for personalized guidance.

Hydration, or the process of maintaining

adequate fluid levels in the body, is essential for overall health and well-being. Water is a fundamental component of our bodies and plays a crucial role in various physiological functions. Here is some ways hydration impacts health:

1. Cellular Function: Water is necessary for basic cellular functions, including transporting nutrients, oxygen, and waste products. Proper hydration ensures that cells can function optimally, leading to improved overall bodily function.

2. Temperature Regulation: Sweating is the body's natural cooling mechanism. When you're dehydrated, your body's ability to regulate temperature can be compromised, potentially leading to overheating and heat-related illnesses.

3. Digestion and Nutrient Absorption: Water is essential for digestion and the absorption of nutrients from the food we consume. It helps break down food in the stomach and aids in the movement of nutrients through the gastrointestinal tract.

4. Joint Lubrication: Adequate hydration supports the lubrication of joints, reducing the risk of joint pain and discomfort. Cartilage, which acts as a cushion between bones, contains a significant amount of water.

5. Cognitive Function: Even mild dehydration can impair cognitive function, leading to difficulties in concentration, memory, and overall mental

performance. Staying hydrated can help maintain optimal brain function.

6. Physical Performance: Whether you're an athlete or engage in regular physical activities, hydration is crucial for performance. Lack of fluids might affect one's strength, coordination, and endurance.

7. Kidney Function: The kidneys play a vital role in filtering waste products and excess substances from the bloodstream. Proper hydration supports kidney function, reducing the risk of kidney stones and other kidney-related issues.

8. Skin Health: Hydrated skin tends to be more elastic and less prone to dryness, flakiness, and wrinkles. Drinking enough water can contribute to maintaining healthy and glowing skin.

9. Mood and Energy Levels: Dehydration can affect mood and energy levels. Feelings of weariness, irritation, and diminished motivation can result from even slight dehydration.

10. Immune System Support: Hydration helps transport immune cells throughout the body, supporting the immune system's ability to fight off infections and illnesses.

11. Detoxification: Water is a key component in the body's natural detoxification processes. It helps flush out waste products and toxins, aiding in the overall health of organs like the liver and colon.

To maintain proper hydration:

- Don't limit your water consumption to times when you're particularly thirsty.

- Monitor your urine color; pale yellow typically indicates adequate hydration.

- Be mindful of your activity level, climate, and individual needs, as they can affect your hydration requirements.

- Eat hydrating foods, such as water-rich fruits and vegetables.

- Limit excessive intake of caffeine, alcohol, and sugary beverages, as they can contribute to dehydration.

Keep in mind that every person has different demands for hydration depending on their age, weight, amount of exercise, and climate. It's important to listen to your body and ensure you're providing it with the fluids it needs to function optimally.

Regular exercise and fitness are essential components of a healthy lifestyle. Engaging in physical activity on a consistent basis offers numerous physical, mental, and emotional benefits. Here's some information about the importance of regular exercise and maintaining fitness:

Physical Benefits:

1. Weight Management: Regular exercise helps to burn calories and maintains a healthy weight. It can also contribute to weight loss when combined with a balanced diet.

2. Cardiovascular Health: Exercise strengthens the heart and improves circulation, reducing the risk of heart diseases. It can lower blood pressure, improve cholesterol levels, and enhance overall cardiovascular function.

3. Muscle Strength and Endurance: Different types of exercises, including strength training and resistance exercises can increase muscle strength and endurance. This not only improves physical performance but also supports joint health.

4. Bone Health: Weight-bearing exercises like walking, running, and strength training can help maintain bone density and reduce the risk of osteoporosis.

5. Flexibility and Balance: Activities like yoga and stretching can enhance flexibility and balance, reducing the risk of injuries from falls and improving overall mobility.

Mental and Emotional Benefits:

1. Stress Reduction: Physical activity triggers the release of endorphins, which are natural mood lifters. Exercise can reduce stress, anxiety, and depression while promoting a positive sense of well-being.

2. Improved Cognitive Function: Regular exercise has been linked to better cognitive function, including enhanced memory, focus, and problem-solving abilities. It may also lower the risk of cognitive decline as you age.

3. Better Sleep: Engaging in regular physical activity can help regulate sleep patterns, leading to improved sleep quality.

4. Boosted Self-Esteem: Achieving fitness goals, such as improved strength or weight loss, can boost self-esteem and confidence.

Tips for Incorporating Regular Exercise:

1. Choose Activities You Enjoy: Find activities that you genuinely enjoy, whether it's running, swimming, dancing, or playing a sport. This makes it more likely that you'll stick with your routine.

2. Set Realistic Goals: Set achievable fitness goals that are specific, measurable, and time-bound. This will give you a sense of purpose and motivation.

3. Gradual Progression: If you're new to exercise, start slowly and gradually increase the intensity and duration of your workouts to avoid injuries.

4. Mix It Up: Use a variety of workouts to work various muscle areas and minimize monotony.

5. Consistency is Key: Aim for regular physical activity. Consistency matters more than occasional

intense workouts.

6. Listen to Your Body: Pay attention to your body's signals. Rest when needed, and don't push yourself too hard, especially if you're feeling unwell or fatigued 6. Listen to Your Body: Pay attention to the cues coming from your body. If you feel sick or exhausted, take the time you need to rest and avoid overexerting yourself.

The goal of regular exercise is to improve your overall health and well-being. It's important to consult a healthcare professional before starting a new exercise program, especially if you have any pre-existing health conditions or concerns.

Cardiovascular activities, often referred to as cardio exercises or aerobic exercises, are physical activities that increase your heart rate and breathing while engaging large muscle groups for an extended period. These activities are essential for maintaining cardiovascular health, improving lung capacity, increasing endurance, and burning calories. Here are some common examples of cardiovascular activities:

1. Running: Running is a popular and effective cardiovascular exercise that can be done outdoors or on a treadmill. It's a high-impact activity that burns a significant amount of calories.

2. Cycling: Whether on a stationary bike or a regular bicycle, cycling is a low-impact exercise that provides an excellent cardiovascular workout.

3. Swimming: Swimming is a low-impact, full-body exercise. It engages multiple muscle groups and promotes cardiovascular fitness.

4. Brisk Walking: Walking at a brisk pace, especially for a sustained period, can be a great cardiovascular activity. It's low-impact and accessible for most fitness levels.

5. Jump Rope: A good approach to get your heart rate up is to jump rope. It improves coordination and works various muscle groups.

6. Dancing: Whether it's formal dance classes or just dancing to your favorite music at home, dancing can be an enjoyable cardiovascular activity.

7. Hiking: Hiking involves walking on trails, often with varying terrains. It not only provides a cardiovascular workout but also allows you to connect with nature.

8. Elliptical Training: Using an elliptical machine at the gym provides a low-impact cardiovascular workout that engages both the upper and lower body.

9. Rowing: Rowing machines provide a full-body workout that strengthens muscles and boosts cardiovascular fitness.

10. High-Intensity Interval Training (HIIT): HIIT involves alternating between intense bursts of exercise and short periods of rest. It is effective at increasing

cardiovascular fitness and calorie burning.

11. Aerobic Classes: Participating in group classes like aerobics, Zumba, or step aerobics can be a fun way to engage in cardiovascular activities.

12. Cross Fit: Cross Fit workouts often include a combination of cardiovascular exercises and strength training, providing a comprehensive fitness routine.

Remember that the intensity, duration, and frequency of cardiovascular activities depend on your fitness level and goals. It's always a good idea to consult a healthcare professional before starting a new exercise regimen, especially if you have any pre-existing health conditions.

Strength training, often known as resistance training or weight training, is a type of exercise that focuses on boosting a person's body's muscular strength and power by applying resistance to the muscles. The resistance can come from various sources, including free weights (like dumbbells and barbells), weight machines, resistance bands, and even bodyweight exercises.

Here are some key aspects and benefits of strength training:

1. Muscle Development: Strength training involves repeatedly contracting muscles against resistance. This leads to the breakdown of muscle fibers, which then repair and grow stronger during the recovery process.

2. Increased Strength: Regular strength training helps increase muscle strength, making everyday tasks easier to perform and improving athletic performance.

3. Bone Health: Strength training can enhance bone density and reduce the risk of osteoporosis, especially when exercises involving weight-bearing are incorporated.

4. Metabolism Boost: Building muscle mass through strength training can help boost metabolism. When at rest, muscle tissue burns more calories than fat tissue, adding to total caloric expenditure.

5. Fat Loss: Strength training, when combined with proper nutrition, can aid in fat loss. As mentioned earlier, increased muscle mass contributes to a higher resting metabolic rate, potentially leading to increased fat burning.

6. Improved Joint Health and Injury Prevention: Strengthening the muscles around joints can enhance stability and reduce the risk of injuries. This is particularly important for those engaged in sports and physical activities.

7. Functional Fitness: Strength training helps improve functional fitness, which means you become better equipped to perform real-life movements and tasks with ease.

8. Mental Health Benefits: Engaging in regular strength training can have positive effects on mental

health by reducing stress, anxiety, and depression.

9. Aesthetic Goals: Many people engage in strength training to achieve a more toned and defined physique.

10. Aging Gracefully: Strength training can counteract age-related muscle loss (sarcopenia) and maintain independence and vitality as you age.

When starting a strength training program, it's important to consider the following:

- Proper Form: Using correct form and technique is crucial to prevent injuries. Consider working with a certified personal trainer, especially when starting out.

- Progressive Overload: To continue seeing results, gradually increase the resistance or intensity of your workouts over time.

- Rest and Recovery: Muscles need time to recover and grow. Be sure to schedule relaxation days into your schedule.

- Balanced Routine: A well-rounded program targets different muscle groups and includes both compound (multi-joint) and isolation (single-joint) exercises.

- Nutrition: Proper nutrition is essential to support muscle growth and recovery. Make sure you're consuming adequate protein and other nutrients.

- Consistency: Like any form of exercise, consistency

is key to seeing results. Aim for a consistent strength-training schedule.

Remember that everyone's fitness goals and starting points are different. Before beginning a new workout regimen, it is wise to speak with a healthcare provider, especially if you have any underlying medical issues. Flexibility and mobility exercises are essential components of a well-rounded fitness routine. They help improve joint range of motion, reduce the risk of injury, enhance posture, and contribute to overall physical well-being. Here are some examples of flexibility and mobility exercises that you can incorporate into your routine:

1. Static Stretching:

These involve holding a stretch for a certain period, usually around 15-30 seconds, without bouncing. Stretches that are frequently performed are hamstring, quad, calf, and shoulder stretches.

2. Dynamic Stretching:

During dynamic stretches, you move your body's parts through their complete range of motion. Arm circles, leg swings, hip circles, and walking lunges are a few examples.

3. Foam Rolling:

Foam rolling, also known as self-myofascial release, uses a foam roller to apply pressure to muscles to release tension and improve mobility. Roll over different muscle groups to target knots and tight spots.

4. Yoga:

Yoga combines flexibility, strength, and balance. Many yoga poses help improve mobility and flexibility, such as downward dog, cobra pose, pigeon pose, and child's pose.

5. Pilates:

Core stability, flexibility, and general body control are the main goals of Pilates. It often involves slow, controlled movements that promote both flexibility and stability.

6. Mobility Drills:

Mobility drills specifically target joint mobility. Examples include shoulder dislocations with a resistance band, hip circles, and wrist circles.

7. Active Isolated Stretching (AIS):

AIS involve holding a stretch for just a couple of seconds and then releasing. This technique can help increase flexibility without triggering the protective stretch reflex.

8. Resistance Band Exercises:

Resistance bands can be used to enhance flexibility

and mobility. For example, you can use a band for shoulder stretches or hip mobility exercises.

9. Tai Chi:

Tai Chi is a martial art that involves slow, flowing movements that can improve balance, flexibility, and relaxation.

10. Calf Raises and Toe Taps:

These exercises target the ankles and calves, helping improve ankle mobility and stability.

When incorporating flexibility and mobility exercises into your routine, keep these tips in mind:

- Warm up first to get the blood flowing to your muscles.

- Exercise in a range of motion without experiencing any pain.

- Breathe deeply and evenly while stretching to relax and enhance the stretch.

- Be consistent. Flexibility and mobility gains come with regular practice over time.

- Listen to your body. If you feel pain or discomfort, stop the exercise and reassess your form.

Remember that everyone's body is different, so it's important to choose exercises that work for you and your level of flexibility. If you have any existing medical conditions or concerns, it's a good idea to consult with a healthcare professional or a fitness expert before starting a new flexibility and mobility routine.

Quality sleep and rest are essential for overall health and well-being. They play a crucial role in maintaining physical, mental, and emotional health. Here's some information about quality sleep and rest:

Quality Sleep:

1. Duration: Adults generally need 7-9 hours of sleep per night, although individual needs can vary. Teenagers and children may need more sleep. Consistently getting enough sleep is important for cognitive function, memory consolidation, and emotional regulation.

2. Sleep Cycles: Sleep consists of cycles of different stages, including rapid eye movement (REM) and non-REM stages. Each cycle takes around 90 minutes and is repeated several times throughout the night. REM sleep is associated with dreaming, while non-REM sleep is further divided into lighter and deeper stages.

3. Sleep Hygiene: Practicing good sleep hygiene can improve the quality of your sleep. This includes maintaining a regular sleep schedule, creating a comfortable sleep environment, avoiding stimulants like caffeine close to bedtime, and engaging in

relaxing activities before sleep.

4. Blue Light Exposure: Exposure to blue light from screens (phones, tablets, and computers) before bedtime can interfere with the production of melatonin, a hormone that regulates sleep. It's recommended to limit screen time at least an hour before sleep or use devices with "night mode" settings that reduce blue light emission.

5. Physical Activity: Regular physical activity can improve sleep quality. However, it's best to avoid intense exercise close to bedtime as it can be stimulating.

6. Caffeine and Alcohol: Consuming caffeine and alcohol close to bedtime can disrupt sleep. These substances can interfere with falling asleep and the quality of sleep during the night.

Rest:

1. Restorative Activities: Rest doesn't only refer to sleep. Engaging in restorative activities during waking hours is also important. This can include relaxation techniques, mindfulness, meditation, deep breathing exercises, and even short breaks during the day.

2. Balancing Work and Rest: It's important to find a balance between work, daily activities, and rest. Overworking or constantly being on the go can lead to burnout and negatively impact your overall health.

3. Mental and Emotional Rest: Rest isn't just about physical relaxation; mental and emotional rest is equally important. Engaging in activities you enjoy, spending time with loved ones, pursuing hobbies, and practicing mindfulness can all contribute to mental and emotional well-being.

4. Quality over Quantity: Just as with sleep, the quality of your waking rest matters. Engaging in activities that truly relax and rejuvenate you will have a more positive impact on your well-being than mere passive time spent without purpose.

In conclusion, both quality sleep and rest are integral to a healthy and balanced life. Prioritizing both aspects can lead to improved physical health, cognitive function, emotional well-being, and overall quality of life.

Sleep is a complex physiological process that consists of different stages and cycles. Sleep stages are distinct phases of sleep characterized by various brain wave patterns and physiological changes. Sleep cycles refer to the progression through these stages during the course of a night's sleep. The two primary types of sleep are rapid eye movement (REM) and non-rapid eye movement (NREM). There are typically four stages of NREM sleep, along with REM sleep. Here's a breakdown of these stages

1. Stage N1 (NREM 1): This is the transition between wakefulness and sleep. During this light sleep stage, your muscles start to relax, and your brain produces

theta waves, which are slower in frequency than wakeful brain waves. This stage is characterized by a relatively easy awakening and might include sensations of falling or floating.

2. Stage N2 (NREM 2): In this stage, your body continues to relax, and your brain waves become more synchronized with occasional bursts of rapid brain activity called sleep spindles. K-complexes, which are large, slow brain waves, also appear. This stage occupies a significant portion of the sleep cycle.

3. Stage N3 (NREM 3): This stage is often referred to as slow-wave sleep (SWS) or deep sleep. It is characterized by slow delta waves on an electroencephalogram (EEG). It's during this stage that your body repairs and regrows tissues, builds bone and muscle, and strengthens the immune system. It can be more difficult to wake up from this stage, and if awakened, you might feel disoriented for a few minutes.

4. REM Sleep: Rapid Eye Movement sleep is a stage where most dreaming occurs. Your brain becomes highly active, similar to wakefulness, and your eyes move rapidly beneath your eyelids. This is when your brain processes emotions, memories, and other cognitive functions. During REM sleep, your body's muscles are mostly paralyzed, which is thought to prevent you from acting out your dreams.

Sleep cycles involve progressing through these stages in a predictable pattern. A typical sleep cycle lasts about 90 minutes and includes multiple cycles throughout the night. As the night progresses, the amount of time spent in REM sleep increases while the time spent in deep NREM sleep (Stage N3) decreases. This is why you might wake up feeling more refreshed in the morning if you wake up after a REM cycle rather than in the middle of a deep sleep cycle.

Understanding sleep stages and cycles is essential for maintaining healthy sleep patterns and addressing sleep-related issues. Devices like sleep trackers and polysomnography (sleep studies) help monitor and analyze these stages to improve sleep quality and overall well-being.

Improving sleep quality is essential for overall well-being and functioning. Here are some suggestions to help you improve the quality of your sleep:

1. Maintain a Consistent Sleep Schedule: Try to go to bed and wake up at the same times every day, even on weekends. This helps regulate your body's internal clock and improve sleep quality over time.

2. Create a Relaxing Bedtime Routine: Engage in calming activities before bed, such as reading, gentle stretching, taking a warm bath, or practicing relaxation techniques like deep breathing or meditation.

3. Limit Exposure to Screens: Reduce exposure to electronic devices (phones, tablets, computers, TVs)

at least an hour before bedtime. Here are some ideas to help you get a better night's sleep:

4. Create a Comfortable Sleep Environment: Make sure your bedroom is conducive to sleep. This includes a comfortable mattress and pillows, appropriate room temperature, and minimal noise and light.

5. Keep an eye on your diet: Stay away from large meals, coffee, and alcohol right before bed. These may impede sleep or make it more difficult to get off to sleep.

6. Exercise Regularly: Regular physical activity can improve sleep quality, but try to finish exercising at least a few hours before bedtime to allow your body to wind down.

7. Manage Stress: Practice stress-reduction techniques during the day, such as exercise, yoga, mindfulness, or deep breathing. Poor sleep can be caused by high amounts of stress.

8. Limit Naps: While short naps can be refreshing, long or late-afternoon naps can interfere with nighttime sleep. If you need to nap, aim for around 20-30 minutes and do so earlier in the day.

9. Monitor Your Intake of Fluids: While hydration is important, try to avoid excessive liquids close to bedtime to minimize nighttime awakenings for bathroom trips.

10. Expose Yourself to Natural Light: Get exposure to natural sunlight during the day, especially in the morning. Natural light helps regulate your body's internal clock and improves sleep-wake cycles.

11. Limit Bedtime Clock-Watching: Constantly checking the clock during the night can increase anxiety about not sleeping, making it even harder to fall asleep. Consider getting out of bed and resting until you feel drowsy if you're having trouble falling asleep.

12. Limit Caffeine and Nicotine: These stimulants can interfere with falling asleep and staying asleep. In the hours before bed, stay away from them.

13. Seek Professional Help: If you've tried these tips and continue to struggle with sleep, consider consulting a healthcare professional. They can help identify underlying issues and provide guidance tailored to your specific situation.

Improving sleep quality takes time and consistency. Implementing these tips gradually and making them a part of your daily routine can have a positive impact on your sleep patterns and overall well-being.

Napping can have several benefits for overall health and well-being. While naps might be associated with laziness or unproductivity, research has shown that strategic and moderate napping can actually enhance cognitive function, mood, and alertness. Here are some potential benefits of napping:

1. Increased Alertness: Short naps, typically lasting around 10 to 20 minutes, can help combat feelings of drowsiness and increase alertness. These brief naps are often referred to as power naps and can provide a quick energy boost without causing grogginess.

2. Improved Cognitive Function: Napping can enhance cognitive functions like memory, learning, and problem-solving. Rapid Eye Movement (REM) sleep, which occurs during longer naps, is associated with memory consolidation and creative thinking.

3. Mood Enhancement: Naps can have positive effects on mood by reducing stress and anxiety. A short nap can help reset your mood and provide a break from the demands of the day.

4. Physical Rejuvenation: Napping can help the body recover from physical fatigue and improve overall physical well-being. It allows your muscles and cells to rest and repair.

5. Boosted Performance: In various studies, napping has been linked to improved performance, especially for tasks that require sustained attention, concentration, and motor skills.

6. Enhanced Learning: Napping can aid in the retention of information learned earlier in the day, as it supports memory consolidation. This is particularly beneficial for students and individuals engaged in

learning-intensive activities.

7. Reduced Sleep Debt: If you didn't get enough sleep the previous night, a nap can help you partially offset the sleep debt, improving your cognitive function and mood until you can get a full night's rest.

8. Cardiovascular Health: Some studies suggest that regular napping may be associated with a reduced risk of cardiovascular events, as it can help lower blood pressure and reduce stress.

Enhancing positivity is crucial for maintaining good mental and emotional well-being. Here are several strategies you can consider incorporating into your life to cultivate a more positive outlook:

1. Practice Gratitude: Regularly take a few moments to reflect on the things you're grateful for. This can help shift your focus away from what's lacking and onto the positive aspects of your life.

2. Positive Affirmations: Use positive affirmations to challenge and overcome self-sabotaging thoughts. Repeat statements that reinforce positive beliefs about yourself and your abilities.

3. Mindfulness and Meditation: Engage in mindfulness and meditation practices to stay present and reduce anxiety. These practices can also help you become more aware of your thought patterns and allow you to respond to negative thoughts in a healthier way.

4. Surround Yourself with Positive People: Hang out with those who inspire and encourage you. Surrounding yourself with positive influences can have a significant impact on your overall outlook.

5. Engage in Physical Activity: Regular exercise has been shown to release endorphins, which are natural mood lifters. Engaging in physical activity can boost your overall sense of well-being.

Make time for enjoyable and relaxing activities. 6. Practice self-care. Whether it's reading, taking a bath, or pursuing a hobby, self-care can contribute to a positive mindset.

7. Limit Negative Influences: Minimize exposure to negative news, toxic relationships, and environments that bring you down. This doesn't mean ignoring problems but being mindful of how much negativity you allow into your life.

8. Focus on Solutions: When faced with challenges, focus on finding solutions rather than dwelling on problems. This shift in mindset can empower you to take action and feel more in control.

9. Celebrate Small Wins: Acknowledge and celebrate even the smallest achievements. This helps build a sense of accomplishment and boosts your self-confidence.

10. Engage in Acts of Kindness: Doing something kind for someone else can create a positive ripple

effect, both in your own mood and in the world around you.

11. Practice Humor: Find humor in everyday situations. Laughter can be a powerful tool for shifting perspective and releasing stress.

12. Set Realistic Goals: Setting achievable goals can give you a sense of purpose and accomplishment. Break larger goals into smaller steps to make them more manageable and celebrate progress along the way.

13. Cultivate Positive Self-Talk: Challenge negative self-talk by questioning its validity and replacing it with more balanced and compassionate thoughts.

14. Learn and Grow: Embrace a growth mindset, viewing challenges as opportunities for learning and growth rather than setbacks.

15. Engage in Activities That Bring Joy: Identify activities that make you feel happy and engaged, and make time for them regularly.

Enhancing positivity is an ongoing process. It's okay to have moments of negativity, but these strategies can help you develop a more optimistic and resilient mindset over time. Try out various strategies to see one suits you the best. However, it's important to note that not all naps are created equal, and there are some potential downsides to consider:

1. Sleep Inertia: Longer naps, especially those lasting more than 30 minutes, can lead to sleep inertia, which is the groggy and disoriented feeling that you experience upon waking up from a deep sleep.

2. Disruption of Nighttime Sleep: Taking excessively long or late-afternoon naps can interfere with your nighttime sleep, leading to difficulties falling asleep or staying asleep at night.

3. Individual Variability: The ideal nap duration and timing can vary from person to person. Some people might feel refreshed after a short nap, while others might need a longer nap to experience the benefits.

To make the most of napping, consider the following tips:

- Keep naps short: A power nap of 10 to 20 minutes is often sufficient to recharge without causing sleep inertia.

- Nap in the early afternoon: Napping too late in the day can affect nighttime sleep. Aim for a nap around mid-afternoon.

- Create a comfortable environment: Find a quiet, dimly lit, and comfortable place to nap.

- Experiment: Pay attention to how different nap durations and timings affect your alertness and mood. Adjust your napping habits accordingly.

In conclusion, when used wisely, napping can be a

valuable tool for enhancing cognitive function, mood, and overall productivity. However, individual preferences and needs vary, so it's important to find a napping routine that works best for you.

CHAPTER THREE

MENTAL AND EMOTIONAL HEALTH

Mental and emotional health is essential aspects of overall well-being. They refer to the state of an individual's psychological and emotional state. Here's a breakdown of these concepts:

1. Mental Health:

Mental health encompasses cognitive, emotional, and social well-being. It relates to how people think, feel, and behave. Good mental health contributes to effective functioning in daily life, healthy relationships, and the ability to cope with challenges. Mental health issues can range from mild to severe and may include conditions like anxiety disorders, depression, bipolar disorder, schizophrenia, and more.

Maintaining good mental health involves factors such as:

- Healthy Coping Mechanisms: Developing healthy ways to manage stress and challenges, such as through exercise, mindfulness, and relaxation techniques.

- Social Support: Building and nurturing supportive relationships with family, friends, and community to provide emotional backup.

- Balanced Lifestyle: Ensuring a balanced routine that includes adequate sleep, a nutritious diet, regular exercise, and engaging in activities that bring joy.

- Seeking Professional Help: Consulting mental health professionals like therapists, counselors, or psychiatrists when needed.

2. Emotional Health:

Emotional health pertains to an individual's ability to recognize, understand, express, and manage their emotions in a healthy way. It involves being in touch with your feelings, having emotional resilience, and having the capacity to handle difficult emotions effectively.

Key components of emotional health include:

- Emotional Awareness: Understanding your own emotions and recognizing their triggers.

- Emotional Regulation: Managing and coping with intense emotions without them overwhelming you or leading to harmful behaviors.

- Empathy: Being able to understand and connect with the emotions of others.

- Positive Relationships: Forming and maintaining healthy relationships that contributes to emotional well-being.

- Self-Care: Practicing activities that promote relaxation, self-compassion, and self-reflection.

Both mental and emotional health is interconnected. Good mental health can contribute to improved emotional health and vice versa. It's important to remember that everyone experiences challenges to their mental and emotional well-being at various points in life. Seeking support when needed and adopting healthy coping strategies are crucial steps in maintaining a positive mental and emotional state.

If you or someone you know is struggling with mental or emotional health issues, it's recommended to reach out to mental health professionals, support groups, or helplines for assistance.

Stress management refers to the techniques and strategies that individuals use to cope with and reduce the negative effects of stress on their mental, emotional, and physical well-being. Stress is a natural response to challenging situations, but chronic or excessive stress can lead to a range of health issues, including anxiety, depression, cardiovascular problems, and more. Effective stress management helps individuals build resilience and maintain a better overall quality of life.

Here are some methods and tactics for reducing stress:

1. Mindfulness and Meditation: Practicing mindfulness and meditation can help you stay present,

reduce anxiety, and manage stress. Techniques like deep breathing, progressive muscle relaxation, and guided imagery can also be effective.

2. Regular Exercise: Engaging in regular physical activity releases endorphins, which are natural mood lifters. Exercise can enhance general health, lower stress, and increase mood.

3. Healthy Lifestyle: A balanced diet, adequate sleep, and avoiding excessive caffeine and alcohol intake can contribute to stress reduction and overall well-being.

4. Time Management: Organizing your tasks, setting priorities, and avoiding procrastination can help you feel more in control and reduce stress related to feeling overwhelmed.

5. Social Support: Talking to friends, family, or a therapist about your feelings can provide emotional support and help you manage stress. Connecting with others and maintaining a support network is important.

6. Relaxation Techniques: Engaging in activities you enjoy, such as reading, listening to music, or spending time in nature, can promote relaxation and reduce stress.

7. Limiting Stressors: Identify and reduce sources of stress where possible. This might involve setting boundaries, saying no to additional commitments, or making lifestyle changes.

8. Problem-Solving: When facing a stressful situation, break it down into smaller steps and develop a plan to address each part. This can make the situation feel more manageable.

9. Humor and Laughter: Finding humor in situations and laughing can help alleviate stress and improve your mood.

10. Creative Outlets: Engaging in creative activities like painting, writing, or playing a musical instrument can provide a positive outlet for emotions and reduce stress.

11. Cognitive Behavioral Therapy (CBT): This therapeutic approach helps individuals identify and change negative thought patterns that contribute to stress and anxiety.

12. Mindset Shift: Cultivate a positive and resilient mindset. Focus on aspects you can control and practice self-compassion.

13. Seek Professional Help: If your stress becomes overwhelming and persistent, consider seeking help from a mental health professional. They can provide guidance and support tailored to your situation.

It's crucial to experiment and discover your personal best because different methods suit different people. Regularly practicing stress management techniques can help you build resilience and better cope with life's challenges.

Stress management refers to a variety of techniques and strategies that individuals can use to cope with and reduce the negative effects of stress on their physical, mental, and emotional well-being. In today's fast-paced world, stress is a common experience that can result from various factors, such as work pressures, personal challenges, health issues, and more. Effective stress management can help improve overall quality of life and prevent stress-related health problems.

Here are some techniques and strategies for managing stress:

1. Identify Stressors: Be aware of your stressors. Once you're aware of what's causing your stress, you can work on addressing or managing those specific factors.

2. Time Management: Organize your tasks and responsibilities. Prioritize what needs to be done, set realistic goals, and avoid overloading yourself.

3. Healthy Lifestyle: Maintain a balanced diet, engage in regular physical activity, and ensure you get enough sleep. These factors contribute to your body's ability to handle stress.

4. Relaxation Techniques: Practice relaxation methods such as deep breathing, meditation, progressive muscle relaxation, or mindfulness. These techniques can help calm your mind and reduce the physiological

effects of stress.

5. Regular Exercise: Physical activity has been shown to reduce stress hormones and increase the release of endorphins, which are natural mood elevators.

6. Social Support: Spend time with friends and loved ones who provide emotional support. It can assist to reduce stress to express your emotions and worries to others.

7. Hobbies and Interests: Engage in activities you enjoy, whether it's reading, painting, playing a musical instrument, or gardening. These activities can serve as a positive distraction from stress.

8. Limit Caffeine and Alcohol: Excessive consumption of caffeine and alcohol can exacerbate feelings of anxiety and stress. Moderation is key.

9. Set Boundaries: Learn to say no when you're overwhelmed with commitments. Setting boundaries helps prevent burnout.

10. Positive Thinking: Practice positive self-talk and focus on gratitude. Cultivating an optimistic mindset can help you approach challenges with a more constructive attitude.

11. Problem-Solving: Break down problems into manageable steps and work on finding solutions. Taking action can give you a sense of control over stressful situations.

12. Seek Professional Help: If your stress becomes overwhelming and starts affecting your daily life, consider seeking support from a therapist, counselor, or mental health professional.

13. Time for Enjoyment: Make time for activities that bring you joy. Laughter and enjoyment have natural stress-reducing effects.

14. Mindfulness and Meditation: Mindfulness involves staying present in the moment without judgment. Meditation practices can help improve focus and reduce stress.

Remember that not all techniques work the same for everyone. It's important to explore different strategies and find what suits you best. Additionally, consistent practice is key to experiencing the full benefits of stress management techniques. If you're struggling with chronic stress or anxiety, don't hesitate to seek professional guidance.

Stress can arise from various sources, and understanding these sources can help individuals manage and mitigate their stress levels. Some common sources of stress include:

1. Workplace Stress: High workloads, tight deadlines, lack of control over tasks, conflicts with coworkers or supervisors, and job insecurity can contribute to workplace stress.

2. Personal Relationships: Problems within personal

relationships, such as conflicts with family members, friends, or romantic partners, can lead to emotional stress.

3. Financial Issues: Financial instability, debt, or struggles to make ends meet can be significant sources of stress.

4. Health Concerns: Personal health issues, chronic illnesses, or concerns about one's health can create stress.

5. Major Life Changes: Events such as moving, divorce, marriage, having a child or the death of a loved one can cause considerable stress.

6. Academic Pressure: Students often experience stress due to academic demands, exams, assignments, and the pressure to perform well.

7. Time Management Challenges: Struggling to balance multiple responsibilities and obligations can lead to stress over time management.

8. Technology and Information Overload: Constant connectivity and exposure to a vast amount of information can lead to stress, especially if there's difficulty in disconnecting.

9. Social Pressure: Societal expectations, cultural norms, and the pressure to conform to certain standards can contribute to stress.

10. Environmental Factors: Living in an environment

with noise, pollution, or other negative factors can impact overall stress levels.

11. Uncertainty and Lack of Control: Feeling uncertain about the future or lacking control over situations can lead to chronic stress.

12. Traumatic Events: Experiencing or witnessing traumatic events, such as accidents, natural disasters, or violence, can result in significant stress.

13. Over commitment: Taking on too many responsibilities or saying yes to too many commitments can lead to feeling overwhelmed and stressed.

14. Perfectionism: Striving for perfection in all areas of life can lead to constant stress and anxiety.

15. Media Exposure: Constant exposure to negative news and media can contribute to stress and a feeling of unease.

It's important to note that individuals may respond differently to these sources of stress, and what one person finds stressful might not be the same for another. Developing effective coping mechanisms, practicing stress management techniques (such as mindfulness, exercise, and relaxation techniques), seeking social support, and, if necessary, consulting with mental health professionals are important steps in managing and reducing stress.

Time management and work-life balance are crucial aspects of maintaining a healthy and productive lifestyle, especially in today's fast-paced world. Effectively managing your time and finding a balance between work and personal life can help reduce stress, increase productivity, and improve overall well-being. Here are some strategies to consider:

1. Set Clear Goals:

Define your short-term and long-term goals, both for work and personal life. Having clear objectives helps you allocate your time and efforts more effectively.

2. Prioritize Tasks:

Identify tasks based on their urgency and importance using methods like the Eisenhower Matrix (quadrants of urgent/important, not urgent/important, urgent/not important, and not urgent/not important).

3. Create a Schedule:

Plan your day or week in advance, allocate specific time blocks for different tasks, including work-related activities, personal activities, exercise, relaxation, and family time.

4. Avoid Multitasking:

Focus on one task at a time. Trying to multitask can result in less productivity and more stress.

5. Use Time Management Tools:

Utilize tools like to-do lists, calendars, and digital apps to keep track of tasks, appointments, and deadlines.

6. Learn to Say No:

Don't overcommit yourself. Politely decline tasks or projects that don't align with your goals or might lead to burnout.

7. Delegate:

Give work to coworkers or family members if at all possible. Your time could be better spent on more crucial tasks as a result.

8. Take Breaks:

Regular breaks during work can actually enhance productivity and mental clarity. Utilize strategies such as the Pomodoro Technique, which involves working for 25 minutes and taking a 5-minute break, to keep your focus.

9. Practice Self-Care:

Prioritize self-care activities such as exercise, meditation, hobbies, and spending time with loved ones. These activities rejuvenate you and contribute to a balanced life.

10. Set Boundaries:

Establish clear boundaries between work and personal life. Don't check work emails or answer business calls in your free time.

11. Flexibility and Adjustments:

Recognize that balance might not always be static. Different life phases might require adjustments in your time allocation.

12. Reflect and Adjust:

Regularly evaluate how you're managing your time and whether your work-life balance is effective. Based on your observations, make the required adjustments.

13. Learn to Disconnect:

In today's digital age, it's important to disconnect from devices and work-related activities to truly relax and recharge.

14. Seek Support:

Talk to friends, family, or mentors about your challenges and goals. They might offer insights or suggestions you haven't considered.

Achieving a perfect balance between work and personal life might be challenging, but the goal is to find a rhythm that works for you and helps you lead a fulfilling and healthy life. It's not just about managing time, but also about managing your energy and priorities.

Mindfulness and self-awareness are concepts often associated with personal growth, well-being, and psychological development. They both involve a heightened level of conscious awareness and understanding of oneself and one's surroundings. While they are related, they have distinct meanings and practices.

1. Mindfulness:

Mindfulness is the practice of being fully present in the moment, paying deliberate attention to your thoughts, feelings, bodily sensations, and the environment without judgment. It entails keeping a detached eye on your feelings and thoughts. Mindfulness is often cultivated through meditation practices, but it can also be applied to everyday activities. It helps in reducing stress, improving focus, and fostering emotional regulation. Mindfulness teaches you to acknowledge whatever is happening without trying to change or control it.

2. Self-Awareness:

Self-awareness refers to having a clear understanding of your own personality, emotions, strengths, weaknesses, beliefs, and motivations. It involves recognizing your thought patterns, behaviors, and reactions in different situations. Self-awareness allows you to recognize when you're acting in alignment with your values and when you're not. It's a fundamental aspect of personal growth and can lead to better decision-making, improved relationships, and a deeper understanding of your own needs and desires.

Practicing mindfulness can lead to increased self-awareness, and vice versa. When you practice mindfulness, you're training yourself to observe your thoughts and feelings with curiosity and without judgment. This process can reveal patterns in your thinking and emotional responses, enhancing your self-awareness. On the other hand, greater self-awareness can aid in being more mindful, as you become more attuned to your thoughts and emotions, making it easier to redirect your focus to the present moment.

Both mindfulness and self-awareness can be developed through various techniques:

- Meditation: Mindfulness meditation involves focusing your attention on your breath or bodily sensations. This helps cultivate present-moment awareness.

- Journaling: Regularly writing in a journal can help you explore your thoughts, emotions, and experiences, leading to increased self-awareness.

- Reflective Practices: Taking time to reflect on your actions, reactions, and choices can provide insights into your behavior and thought patterns.

- Mindful Activities: Engaging fully in activities like walking, eating, or even washing dishes, while paying full attention to the sensory experiences involved, can promote mindfulness.

- Feedback from Others: Seeking feedback from trusted friends, mentors, or therapists can offer an external perspective on your behavior and tendencies.

Developing mindfulness and self-awareness takes time and consistent effort. It's a journey of self-discovery that can lead to greater emotional resilience, improved relationships, and a more fulfilled life.

Practicing mindfulness involves cultivating a state of nonjudgmental awareness of the present moment. It can be done through formal meditation sessions or by integrating mindfulness into your daily activities. Here's a step-by-step guide to get you started with mindfulness practice:

1. Find a Quiet Space:

Select a place that is peaceful and comfortable and where you won't be bothered. Lie down or sit with a relaxed but attentive posture.

2. Focus on Your Breath:

Take a few relaxing breaths while closing your eyes. Allow your breath to settle back into its regular rhythm after that. As you breathe in and out, pay close attention to how it feels. You can focus on the rise and fall of your chest or the feeling of your breath at the nostrils.

3. Be Present:

Thoughts and diversion may surface as you concentrate on your breathing. This is natural. Instead of trying to suppress these thoughts, simply acknowledge them and gently redirect your attention back to your breath. You're educating your mind to come back to the present.

4. Nonjudgmental Awareness:

As you continue to breathe and observe, practice nonjudgmental awareness. This entails paying attention to your feelings, ideas, and experiences without judging them as positive or negative. Just notice them as they come and go.

5. Body Scan:

Another approach is the body scan. Gradually shift your attention from your breath to different parts of your body, starting from your toes and moving upward. Notice any sensations, tensions, or feelings without trying to change them.

6. Open Awareness:

You can also practice open awareness, where you expand your awareness to include all sensory experiences – sounds, physical sensations, thoughts, and emotions. Allow everything to be present in your awareness without focusing on any one thing.

7. Practice Regularly:

Consistency is key. Start with brief sessions of 5 to 10 minutes, and as you get more at ease, progressively lengthen them. Aim for daily practice.

8. Apply Mindfulness to Daily Activities:

Extend mindfulness beyond formal meditation sessions. Engage in your daily activities mindfully. Pay full attention to what you're doing, whether it's eating, walking, or even brushing your teeth.

9. Be Patient:

Mindfulness is a skill that takes time to develop. Be patient with yourself and avoid self-criticism. It's normal for your mind to wander; the practice is in gently bringing it back.

10. Seek Guidance:

If you're new to mindfulness, you might find it helpful to use guided mindfulness meditation apps or videos. These can provide structure and guidance as you learn the practice.

Remember, mindfulness is a lifelong journey. The goal is not to achieve a particular state but to develop a more compassionate and present relationship with yourself and the world around you. Over time, you'll likely notice the benefits in your overall well-being, stress reduction, and ability to navigate life's challenges with greater clarity.

Cultivating emotional intelligence (EI) involves developing a set of skills and abilities that enable you to recognize, understand, manage, and effectively use your own emotions, as well as understand and influence the emotions of others. Emotional intelligence plays a crucial role in personal and professional success, as it contributes to effective communication, strong relationships, and overall well-being. Here are steps to help you cultivate emotional intelligence:

1. Self-Awareness:

- Recognize Your Emotions: Pay attention to your feelings as they arise throughout the day. Identify and label them accurately.

- Reflect on Triggers: Understand what situations, people, or events trigger specific emotions in you. This helps you anticipate and manage your responses.

2. Self-Regulation:

- Practice Emotional Regulation: Learn to manage your emotions rather than letting them control you. Techniques like deep breathing, mindfulness, and meditation can help.

- Pause before Reacting: When faced with a strong emotion, take a moment to pause before responding.

This allows you to choose a thoughtful response rather than reacting impulsively.

3. Motivation:

- Set Meaningful Goals: Identify goals that genuinely motivate you. Having a clear sense of purpose fuels your motivation.

- Develop a growth mindset by viewing obstacles as chances for improvement. See setbacks as learning experiences.

4. Empathy:

-Practice Active Listening: Truly listen to others without interrupting or planning your response. Focus on understanding their perspective.

- Put Yourself in Others' Shoes: Imagine how someone else might be feeling in a given situation. This helps you connect with their emotions.

5. Social Skills:

- Develop Effective Communication: Learn to express your thoughts and feelings clearly and respectfully. Be an attentive and empathetic listener.

- Resolve Conflicts: Practice resolving conflicts in a constructive manner. Instead of assigning blame, concentrate on finding solutions.

6. Continuous Learning:

- Reflect on Interactions: Regularly reflect on your interactions and emotions. Think about what went well and where you can make improvements.

- Seek Feedback: Ask for feedback from trusted individuals to gain insights into how you come across emotionally.

7. Mindfulness Practice:

- Cultivate Present-Moment Awareness: Engage in mindfulness meditation to enhance your awareness of emotions as they arise without judgment.

- Observe Thoughts and Feelings: Mindfulness helps you observe your thoughts and feelings without being consumed by them.

8. Develop Resilience:

- Adapt to Change: Embrace change and uncertainty as opportunities to learn and grow. Being resilient enables you to recover from setbacks.

9. Practice Empathetic Leadership:

- Lead with Empathy: If you're in a leadership role, focus on understanding the emotions and needs of your team members.

10. Embrace Diversity and Inclusion:

- Appreciate Differences: Recognize and appreciate the emotional diversity among people from different backgrounds and cultures.

Remember that cultivating emotional intelligence is an ongoing process that requires dedication and self-reflection. By consciously working on these skills, you can enhance your ability to navigate emotions, build stronger relationships, and create a more harmonious and successful life both personally and professionally.

Journaling offers a range of psychological, emotional, and even physical benefits. Here are a few of the main benefits of keeping a journal:

1. Emotional Expression: Journaling provides a safe and private space to express your thoughts, feelings, and emotions without fear of judgment. This can help you process complex emotions, reduce stress, and enhance emotional well-being.

2. Stress Reduction: Writing about your worries, anxieties, and stresses can help release the mental burden and reduce their impact on your overall well-being. It's a way to externalize your thoughts and gain perspective on your challenges.

3. Clarity and Self-Discovery: Journaling encourages self-reflection and self-awareness. Through the act of writing, you can gain insights into your own thoughts, behaviors, and patterns, which can lead to personal growth and a better understanding of yourself.

4. Goal Setting and Achievement: Writing down your goals, aspirations, and plans can make them more

concrete and achievable. Regularly journaling about your progress can help you stay accountable and track your achievements over time.

5. Problem Solving: Journaling allows you to analyze and dissect problems in a structured manner. Writing about challenges you're facing can help you brainstorm solutions and make more informed decisions.

6. Creativity Boost: Keeping a journal can stimulate your creativity by providing an outlet for free-form expression. You can experiment with new ideas, sketch, doodle, or jot down inspirations that come to you.

7. Memory Enhancement: Writing about your experiences, whether they're everyday moments or significant events, helps solidify memories. Looking back at your journal can evoke vivid recollections of the past.

8. Gratitude and Positivity: Practicing gratitude by writing about positive experiences, accomplishments, or things you're thankful for can improve your overall mood and outlook on life.

9. Catharsis: Journaling can be cathartic, allowing you to release pent-up emotions and feelings. It can serve as a therapeutic tool to process trauma or challenging experiences.

10. Self-Care: Taking time to sit down and write in a

journal can be an act of self-care. It provides a quiet, reflective space for you to focus on yourself and your well-being.

11. Improvement in Communication Skills: Regular writing in a journal can enhance your writing skills, which can have positive effects on your ability to communicate effectively in various areas of life.

12. Time Management: Planning and recording daily tasks, events, and reflections in a journal can help improve your time management and organizational skills.

13. Record of Progress: Your journal can serve as a record of your personal journey, allowing you to track your growth, development, and changing perspectives over time.

Positive psychology is a field of psychology that focuses on the study of positive emotions, strengths, virtues, and factors that contribute to human well-being and flourishing. One of the central themes of positive psychology is the pursuit of happiness. Here's how positive psychology relates to happiness:

1. Shift from Pathology to Well-Being: Traditional psychology often focused on addressing mental illness and negative aspects of human behavior. Positive psychology, however, emphasizes studying and promoting the positive aspects of human functioning

to enhance overall well-being.

2. Subjective Well-Being: Positive psychology places a strong emphasis on subjective well-being, which includes life satisfaction, positive emotions, and a sense of purpose and meaning in life. Researchers aim to understand what factors contribute to individuals' sense of happiness and fulfillment.

3. Personal Strengths and Virtues: Positive psychology places a strong emphasis on discovering and developing one's personal strengths and virtues. By focusing on strengths like gratitude, kindness, resilience, and creativity, individuals can lead more fulfilling lives and experience greater happiness.

4. Positive Emotions: Positive psychology studies the effects of positive emotions such as joy, gratitude, contentment, and love. Cultivating these emotions can enhance overall life satisfaction and contribute to a more positive outlook.

5. Flow and Engagement: Positive psychology explores the concept of "flow," which is a state of deep engagement and absorption in an activity. Experiencing flow contributes to happiness by providing a sense of accomplishment and fulfillment.

6. Resilience and Coping: Positive psychology acknowledges that challenges and setbacks are a part of life. It focuses on developing resilience, the ability to bounce back from adversity, as a key factor in maintaining happiness and well-being.

7. Gratitude and Mindfulness: Practices like gratitude journaling and mindfulness meditation, often promoted in positive psychology, have been shown to increase feelings of happiness and well-being. They encourage individuals to focus on the present moment and appreciate the positive aspects of life.

8. Positive Relationships: Positive psychology emphasizes the importance of social connections and positive relationships for happiness. Strong social support networks contribute to emotional well-being and life satisfaction.

9. Purpose and Meaning: Finding a sense of purpose and meaning in life is a central component of happiness. Positive psychology explores how individuals can discover and pursue meaningful goals that contribute to their well-being.

10. Cultivating Positive Experiences: Positive psychology encourages individuals to engage in activities that bring them joy and fulfillment, whether that's pursuing hobbies, spending time with loved ones, or contributing to their community.

In essence, positive psychology seeks to provide individuals with tools and insights to lead more fulfilling lives by focusing on their strengths, positive emotions, and factors that contribute to overall well-being and happiness. It's important to note that while negative emotions and challenges are a natural part of life, positive psychology provides a framework for enhancing the positive aspects of human experience.

The science of positive emotions is a branch of psychology and neuroscience that focuses on understanding the nature, causes, effects, and mechanisms of positive emotional experiences. Positive emotions are those feelings and states that contribute to an individual's well-being, happiness, and overall positive psychological functioning. They play a crucial role in enhancing mental health, resilience, and quality of life.

Key concepts and areas within the science of positive emotions include:

1. Emotion Theory: Positive emotions are typically considered to be discrete emotional states that are characterized by pleasant feelings, such as joy, gratitude, contentment, and love. These emotions are distinct from negative emotions like sadness, anger, and fear.

2. Broaden-and-Build Theory: This theory, proposed by psychologist Barbara Fredrickson, suggests that positive emotions broaden an individual's thought-action repertoire, promoting creativity, open-mindedness, and cognitive flexibility. Over time, this broadened mindset contributes to building psychological resources, resilience, and personal growth.

3. Positive Psychology: Positive psychology is a larger movement within psychology that emphasizes studying human strengths, virtues, and well-being, rather than solely focusing on psychological disorders.

Positive emotions are a fundamental aspect of positive psychology, as they contribute to flourishing and thriving in life.

4. Neuroscience of Positive Emotions: Neuroscientists study the brain regions and neural pathways associated with positive emotions. Research using brain imaging techniques such as functional magnetic resonance imaging (fMRI) has identified areas like the prefrontal cortex and the reward circuitry as being involved in positive emotional experiences.

5. Positive Emotion Regulation: Understanding how individuals regulate their positive emotions is an important aspect of this field. Effective emotion regulation strategies contribute to maintaining and enhancing positive emotional experiences.

6. Benefits of Positive Emotions: Positive emotions have been linked to numerous psychological and physiological benefits. They can enhance overall well-being, buffer against stress, improve physical health, and strengthen social connections.

7. Positive Emotions and Relationships: Positive emotions play a critical role in forming and maintaining positive relationships. Expressing positive emotions like gratitude and empathy can strengthen social bonds and create a positive social environment.

8. Cultural Variations: Positive emotional experiences can be influenced by cultural norms and practices.

Different cultures may emphasize certain positive emotions more than others, leading to variations in how individuals experience and express them.

9. Interventions and Practices: Researchers and therapists often develop interventions and practices aimed at promoting positive emotions and well-being. These may include gratitude exercises, mindfulness meditation, acts of kindness, and other activities that foster positive emotional states.

10. Subjective Well-Being: Positive emotions are closely tied to subjective well-being, which refers to an individual's overall evaluation of their life satisfaction and happiness. Positive emotions contribute significantly to an individual's overall sense of well-being.

Studying positive emotions contributes to a more holistic understanding of human emotions and behavior, and it has implications for various fields, including psychology, education, healthcare, and personal development.

Gratitude refers to the practice of recognizing and appreciating the positive aspects of one's life, experiences, and relationships. It involves acknowledging the good things that we have, rather than focusing on what we lack or desire. The impact of gratitude on well-being is well-documented and encompasses various psychological, emotional, and even physical benefits. Here's how gratitude can positively influence well-being:

1. Positive Emotions: Expressing gratitude often leads to an increase in positive emotions such as happiness, joy, and contentment. When you focus on the things you're grateful for, you naturally shift your attention away from negative thoughts and feelings.

2. Stress Reduction: Gratitude can help lower stress levels by promoting a positive outlook and reducing feelings of anxiety. When you're thankful for the good things in your life, it becomes easier to manage challenges and setbacks.

3. Improved Mental Health: Practicing gratitude has been linked to lower rates of depression and improved mental well-being. It can help shift your perspective from dwelling on problems to focusing on the positive aspects of life.

4. Enhanced Relationships: Expressing gratitude can strengthen interpersonal relationships. When you show appreciation for others, it fosters a sense of connection, trust, and mutual respect.

5. Increased Resilience: Grateful individuals tend to exhibit greater resilience in the face of adversity. They are more likely to find meaning and lessons in challenging situations, which aids in coping and personal growth.

6. Better Physical Health: Gratitude has been associated with improved physical health outcomes, including better sleep, reduced blood pressure, and a stronger immune system. Positive emotions from

gratitude can have a direct impact on the body's physiological processes.

7. Boosted Self-Esteem: Recognizing the positive aspects of your life can boost your self-esteem and self-worth. This, in turn, contributes to greater overall life satisfaction.

8. Mindfulness and Present Moment Awareness: Gratitude encourages you to be more mindful and present in your daily life. When you're appreciating the present moment and what it offers, you're less likely to get caught up in worries about the past or future.

9. Altered Perspective on Challenges: Gratitude helps you reframe challenges and setbacks. Instead of viewing them as insurmountable obstacles, you're more likely to see them as opportunities for growth and learning.

10. Generosity and Altruism: Gratitude can inspire a desire to give back and help others. When you recognize how fortunate you are, you may be more inclined to support those who are less fortunate.

To incorporate gratitude into your life and experience its benefits, consider keeping a gratitude journal, regularly expressing appreciation to loved ones, practicing mindfulness, and taking time to reflect on the positive aspects of each day. By cultivating gratitude, you can enhance your overall well-being and create a more positive and fulfilling life

CHAPTER FOUR

SOCIAL WELL-BEING

Social well-being refers to the quality and state of an individual's social relationships, interactions, and overall sense of belonging within their community and society. It is one of the dimensions of well-being that encompasses an individual's ability to maintain positive and fulfilling relationships, engage in meaningful social activities, and feel a sense of connection and support from others.

Social well-being is often considered an essential component of overall well-being and is closely linked to psychological, emotional, and physical health. A strong social support network can provide emotional comfort, practical assistance, and a sense of purpose, which can contribute to improved mental and physical health outcomes.

Factors that contribute to social well-being include:

1. Social Connections: Building and maintaining positive relationships with family, friends, colleagues, and community members.

2. Community Involvement: Participating in social and community activities that align with one's interests and values.

3. Sense of Belonging: Feeling accepted, valued, and

connected to a group or community.

4. Communication Skills: Effective communication and interpersonal skills that foster healthy interactions and relationships.

5. Empathy and Compassion: Being able to understand and share the feelings of others, leading to more meaningful connections.

6. Supportive Relationships: Having people who provide emotional, practical, and instrumental support during challenging times.

7. Respect and Dignity: Treating and being treated with respect, consideration, and kindness.

Promoting social well-being involves nurturing positive relationships, maintaining a healthy work-life balance, engaging in social activities, and seeking help when needed. Strong social connections can help individuals cope with stress, reduce feelings of loneliness and isolation, and contribute to a greater sense of happiness and life satisfaction.

It's important to note that social well-being can vary greatly from person to person, and cultural, societal, and personal factors play a significant role in shaping an individual's experiences and perceptions of social well-being.

Building a healthy relationship is a multifaceted process that requires effort, communication, trust, and understanding from both individuals involved. Whether it's a romantic relationship, a friendship, or a family relationship, here are some key principles to consider:

1. Clear and honest communication is the cornerstone of any successful partnership. Talk to one another about your ideas, emotions, and worries. Listen actively and without judgment. Be open to talking about difficult subjects and avoid making assumptions.

2. Respect: Be respectful and considerate to one another.

Acknowledge each other's feelings, opinions, and boundaries. Respect each other's individuality and differences.

3. Trust: Trust is vital in any relationship. Be reliable, keep your promises, and be consistent in your actions. If trust has been broken, work together to rebuild it through transparency and consistency.

4. Quality Time: Spend quality time together to nurture your bond. Engage in activities you both enjoy, and make an effort to connect emotionally and intellectually.

5. Support: Be each other's support system. Celebrate accomplishments and provide solace in trying circumstances. Show empathy and be willing to provide a listening ear.

6. Healthy Boundaries: Establish clear boundaries to maintain individual autonomy and protect the relationship. Respect each other's personal space, opinions, and needs.

7. Conflict Resolution: Disagreements are normal, but how you handle those matters. Focus on resolving conflicts constructively, rather than trying to "win" an argument. Practice active listening and find compromise.

8. Empathy and Understanding: Try to understand each other's perspectives and feelings. Put yourself in the other person's shoes to better grasp their emotions and motivations.

9. Appreciation and Gratitude: Express appreciation for each other regularly. Acknowledge the positive qualities and efforts your partner brings to the relationship.

10. Shared Values and Goals: Having common values, goals, and interests can help strengthen the bond between you. It gives you a sense of purpose and direction as a couple.

11. Space for Individual Growth: Encourage each other's personal growth and pursuits. A healthy relationship allows space for both individuals to continue evolving and pursuing their passions.

12. Apologize and Forgive: Be willing to apologize when you're wrong, and forgive each other's mistakes.

Holding onto grudges can damage the relationship over time.

13. Intimacy: Emotional, physical, and intellectual intimacy all contribute to a well-rounded connection. Communicate your needs and desires openly, while respecting each other's comfort zones.

14. Teamwork: Approach challenges as a team. Collaborate on decision-making and problem-solving to demonstrate that you're in this together.

15. Patience: Building a healthy relationship takes time. Be patient and give the relationship room to develop naturally.

Remember that no relationship is perfect, and it's normal to encounter challenges. The key is to face these challenges together with mutual respect, understanding, and a willingness to grow both as individuals and as a couple. If issues become overwhelming or persistent, seeking guidance from a relationship counselor or therapist can be beneficial.

Nurturing friendships and connections is essential for maintaining meaningful and fulfilling relationships in your life. Here are some tips to help you foster and strengthen those connections:

1. Effective Communication: Open and honest communication is the foundation of any strong

relationship. Listen actively, express your thoughts and feelings clearly, and show empathy towards your friends' experiences.

2. Quality Time: Spend quality time together, whether it's in person, through video calls, or even messaging. Engage in activities you both enjoy, which can help create lasting memories.

3. Show Appreciation: Express gratitude for your friends' presence in your life. Small gestures like sending a heartfelt message, giving compliments, or offering to help can go a long way in showing you value the relationship.

4. Be Reliable: Consistency is key. When your friends need you, be there for them, and keep your promises. Reliability builds trust and demonstrates your dedication to the friendship.

5. Respect Differences: Friends may have different opinions, interests, and lifestyles. Accept these variations and learn from one another. A diverse group of friends can provide valuable perspectives and enrich your experiences.

6. Supportive Environment: Create a safe and supportive space where your friends feel comfortable sharing their thoughts and emotions without fear of judgment. Be a good listener and offer advice when appropriate.

7. Celebrate Achievements: Celebrate your friends'

successes and milestones, whether big or small. Sharing in their joy and acknowledging their achievements helps strengthen the bond between you.

8. Forgive and Apologize: No relationship is without its conflicts or misunderstandings. Be ready to forgive and apologize when needed. Address conflicts calmly and respectfully, to find resolutions together.

9. Maintain Balance: While friendships are important, it's also essential to maintain a healthy balance between your social life and other commitments. This balance ensures you're able to give time to your friends while also taking care of yourself.

10. Be Patient: Friendships evolve over time. Some friendships may require more effort than others, and that's okay. Be patient and understanding as relationships naturally change and grow.

11. Stay Connected: In our busy lives, it's easy for friendships to fade due to lack of contact. Make an effort to stay in touch regularly, even if it's just a quick check-in or a shared meme.

12. Respect Boundaries: Understand and respect each other's boundaries. Everyone has their limits, and acknowledging them shows that you care about their comfort and well-being.

Remember that nurturing friendships is a two-way street. Both parties need to contribute effort and care to maintain a strong connection. As you invest in your friendships, you'll find that they bring joy, support, and a sense of belonging to your life.

Effective communication skills are essential for successfully conveying information, ideas, thoughts, and emotions to others in a clear, understandable, and impactful manner. Whether in personal, professional, or social contexts, strong communication skills can significantly enhance relationships, collaboration, and overall effectiveness. Here are some key components of effective communication skills:

1. Clarity: Deliver your message in a clear and concise manner. Use simple language and avoid jargon or complex vocabulary that could confuse the listener.

2. Active Listening: Pay close attention to the speaker, showing that you are engaged and interested. This involves maintaining eye contact, nodding, and avoiding interruptions. Respond appropriately to show you understand and are actively processing what's being said.

3. Empathy: Understand and acknowledge the emotions and perspectives of the other person. This helps build rapport and shows that you care about their feelings and point of view.

4. Nonverbal Communication: Body language, facial expressions, gestures, and tone of voice play a crucial role in communication. Be aware of these cues to

ensure that your verbal and nonverbal messages align.

5. Respect: Show respect for the other person's opinions and ideas, even if you disagree. Treat others with courtesy and avoid using disrespectful language or behaviors.

6. Openness and Honesty: Be transparent and truthful in your communication. Avoid misleading or concealing information, as this can erode trust.

7. Feedback: Provide constructive feedback and be receptive to receiving feedback from others. This promotes growth and improvement in communication and relationships.

8. Adaptability: Tailor your communication style to the preferences and needs of your audience. Different strategies could be necessary depending on the scenario and the person.

9. Asking Questions: Ask relevant and open-ended questions to encourage deeper conversations and demonstrate your interest in the topic.

Community engagement and support refer to the processes and activities that involve connecting with and assisting individuals within a specific community. These efforts aim to foster a sense of belonging, encourage participation, and provide resources or assistance to meet the needs of community members. Community engagement and support are essential in various contexts, including neighborhoods, online communities, non-profit organizations, educational institutions, and more.

Key aspects of community engagement and support include:

1. Building Relationships: Establishing meaningful connections with community members by understanding their interests, concerns, and aspirations. This can be achieved through open communication, active listening, and regular interactions.

2. Encouraging Participation: Encouraging community members to actively contribute, collaborate, and participate in community activities, events, and discussions. This involvement helps build a sense of ownership and belonging.

3. Providing Resources: Offering resources, information, and tools that address the needs and challenges faced by the community. This could involve workshops, training sessions, educational materials, and access to essential services.

4. Creating Inclusive Spaces: Creating environments that are welcoming and inclusive for all members, regardless of their backgrounds, identities, or abilities. Fostering a sense of equity and diversity is crucial for building a strong and resilient community.

5. Problem Solving: Identifying and addressing issues or concerns within the community, whether they're

related to infrastructure, safety, or social issues. Collaborative problem-solving can strengthen community bonds.

6. Empowerment: Empowering individuals within the community to take leadership roles, make decisions, and contribute to the overall growth and development of the community.

7. Communication Platforms: Utilizing various communication channels such as social media, community websites, newsletters, and forums to keep members informed about events, news, and opportunities for engagement.

8. Feedback and Evaluation: Regularly seeking feedback from community members to assess the effectiveness of engagement efforts and identify areas for improvement. Continuous evaluation ensures that strategies remain relevant and responsive to evolving needs.

9. Partnerships: Collaborating with other organizations, local authorities, businesses, and institutions to leverage resources and expertise that can benefit the community.

10. Long-Term Sustainability: Developing strategies that ensure the ongoing sustainability of community engagement and support initiatives, even as the community evolves over time.

Effective community engagement and support

contribute to a stronger sense of community identity, improved well-being, and the development of social networks that can enhance resilience and problem-solving capabilities. Whether it's a physical neighborhood or an online platform, creating a culture of collaboration and mutual support is essential for building thriving communities.

10. Organization: Structure your communication logically, using an introduction, main points, and a conclusion. This makes it easier for your audience to follow your message.

11. Conflict Resolution: Develop skills to handle disagreements and conflicts in a respectful and constructive manner. Instead of placing blame, concentrate on finding solutions.

12. Cultural Sensitivity: Be aware of cultural differences in communication styles, norms, and customs. This helps you avoid misunderstandings and promotes effective cross-cultural communication.

13. Use of Technology: In today's digital age, being proficient in various communication tools (email, social media, video conferencing, etc.) is important for effective communication.

14. Practice: Like any skill, effective communication requires practice. Regularly engage in conversations, presentations, and interactions to refine your skills.

15. Confidence Believe in the value of your message

and convey it with confidence. However, avoid coming across as arrogant or overly assertive.

Remember that effective communication is a two-way street. While working on your communication skills is important, being receptive to others' communication efforts and adjusting your approach based on their feedback is equally vital.

Setting boundaries and practicing assertiveness are important skills for maintaining healthy relationships, managing stress, and advocating for your own needs and well-being. Here's a breakdown of both concepts and some tips on how to effectively implement them:

1. Setting Boundaries:

Boundaries are the limits you establish between yourself and others to protect your physical, emotional, and mental well-being. They help you define what is acceptable and what isn't in your interactions with others. Setting clear boundaries can prevent feelings of being overwhelmed, taken advantage of, or disrespected.

Tips for Setting Boundaries:

- Know Your Limits: Reflect on your values, needs, and feelings to identify where you need boundaries.

- Be Clear and Specific: Clearly communicate your boundaries to others in a respectful and straightforward manner.

- Use "I" Statements: Express your needs using statements like "I feel uncomfortable when..." or "I need some space to..."

- Practice Self-Awareness: Pay attention to how you feel in different situations to recognize when your boundaries are being crossed.

- Start Small: Begin with smaller boundaries and gradually work your way up to more complex ones.

- Stay Consistent: Enforce your boundaries consistently to establish a pattern that others can understand and respect.

2. Assertiveness:

Assertiveness involves expressing your thoughts, feelings, and needs in a direct and respectful way, while considering the rights and feelings of others. It's a balanced communication style that helps you stand up for yourself without being aggressive or passive.

Tips for Practicing Assertiveness:

- Use Clear Communication: Express your thoughts and needs clearly, using a confident tone and body language.

- Practice Active Listening: Pay attention to what others are saying, and respond thoughtfully rather than reacting impulsively.

- Use "I" Statements: State your feelings and needs using phrases like "I think," "I feel," or "I would like."

- Be Open to Compromise: Consider the needs of others and be open to finding solutions that benefit everyone.

- Stay Calm: Maintain a calm demeanor, even if the conversation becomes challenging. Refrain from yelling or acting defensively.

- Stand Your Ground: If someone challenges your boundaries or needs, calmly reassert them while maintaining respect.

Remember:

- Setting boundaries and practicing assertiveness might feel uncomfortable at first, especially if you're not used to it. However, these skills improve with practice.

- Building healthy relationships requires mutual respect for each other's boundaries and needs.

- It's okay to prioritize your well-being and needs without feeling guilty.

- Not everyone will respond positively to your boundaries or assertiveness, but that doesn't diminish their importance.

Ultimately, both setting boundaries and practicing assertiveness are about building healthier relationships and fostering better communication. These skills can lead to increased self-confidence, reduced stress, and more fulfilling interactions with others.

Finding like-minded communities can be a rewarding way to connect with people who share your interests, passions, and values. Here are some strategies to help you find and join such communities:

1. Online Platforms:

  - Social Media: Platforms like Facebook, Reddit, and Twitter have numerous groups and communities dedicated to various topics. Use hash tags or search keywords to find relevant groups.

  - Forums and Discussion Boards: Websites like Reddit, Quora, Stack Exchange, and specialized forums cater to specific interests and hobbies.

  - Meet up: This platform helps you find local groups that gather for various activities, events, and discussions.

2. Niche Websites:

  - Search for websites that focus on your particular interest. Blogs, forums, and websites dedicated to specific topics often have vibrant communities.

3. Attend Events:

  - Conferences, seminars, workshops, and local events related to your interests can be excellent places to meet like-minded people in person.

4. Local Groups:

- Check for clubs, organizations, or hobby groups in your local area. Libraries, community centers, and bulletin boards might have information about these groups.

5. Volunteer Opportunities:

- Engaging in volunteer work related to your interests can lead you to individuals who share your values and passions.

6. Classes and Workshops:

- Enroll in classes or workshops that align with your interests. These can be related to arts, crafts, sports, fitness, technology, or any other field you're passionate about.

7. Online Courses:

- Platforms like Coursera, Udemy, and Khan Academy offer online courses where you can interact with other learners who share your interests.

8. Book Clubs:

- If you enjoy reading, consider joining a book club that focuses on your preferred genre or authors.

9. Gaming Communities:

- If you're into gaming, there are numerous online gaming communities, forums, and platforms where gamers gather to discuss and play together.

10. Interest-Specific Apps:

- Some mobile apps are designed to connect people with specific interests, such as fitness, language learning, photography, and more.

11. Professional Networks:

- LinkedIn and industry-specific websites can help you connect with like-minded professionals in your field.

12. Hobby Stores and Events:

-Visit stores related to your hobbies and inquire about any events or gatherings they might host.

When joining these communities, remember to be respectful, open-minded, and willing to contribute positively. It's important to participate actively and genuinely engage with others to build meaningful connections.

Volunteering and giving back to the community are important ways to make a positive impact on the world around you. It involves contributing your time, skills, or resources to help others, organizations, or causes without expecting monetary compensation. Here's some information to consider about volunteering and giving back:

Benefits of Volunteering and Giving Back:

1. Personal Satisfaction: Volunteering can bring a sense of fulfillment and happiness as you see the direct impact of your efforts on individuals and communities.

2. Skill Development: Volunteering provides opportunities to learn new skills, enhance existing ones, and gain practical experience that could benefit your personal and professional growth.

3. Networking: Volunteering can help you connect with people who share your interests and values, potentially leading to new friendships and networking opportunities.

4. Improved Mental Health: Engaging in acts of kindness and helping others has been linked to improved mental well-being and reduced stress levels.

5. Community Building: Volunteering strengthens local communities and fosters a sense of unity and shared responsibility among residents.

6. Positive Example: Your involvement can inspire others to give back, creating a ripple effect of kindness and generosity.

Ways to Give Back:

1. Volunteer for Nonprofits: Numerous nonprofit organizations rely on volunteers to carry out their missions. You can contribute your time by assisting with events, programs, fundraising, administrative tasks, and more.

2. Mentorship and Tutoring: Share your knowledge and expertise by mentoring individuals or tutoring students who could benefit from your guidance.

3. Supporting Vulnerable Populations: Volunteer at shelters, food banks, hospitals, or nursing homes to provide assistance to those in need, such as the homeless, elderly, or sick.

4. Environmental Conservation: Participate in initiatives to protect the environment, such as clean-up events, tree planting, and wildlife preservation.

5. Virtual Volunteering: Many opportunities allow you to contribute remotely, such as online tutoring, content creation, or social media management for nonprofit organizations.

6. Skill-Based Volunteering: Offer your professional skills, such as graphic design, writing, marketing, or legal expertise, to help organizations meet their needs.

7. Donations: While volunteering involves giving your time, donating money, goods, or resources to charitable organizations is another impactful way to give back.

Getting Started:

1. Identify Your Passion: Choose a cause or organization that aligns with your interests and values. You'll be more motivated to contribute if you're passionate about the work.

2. Research Opportunities: Look for local charities, nonprofits, or community centers that need volunteers. Websites like Volunteer Match, Idealist, and local volunteer centers can help you find opportunities.

3. Assess Your Availability: Determine how much time you can commit to volunteering. It's important to find a balance that works for you.

4. Contact Organizations: Reach out to organizations to inquire about volunteer opportunities and their application process.

5. Start Small: If you're new to volunteering, begin with shorter-term commitments to gauge your interest and availability.

6. Stay Committed: Once you've started volunteering, try to stay consistent and reliable. The impact you make can grow over time.

Remember that giving back is a personal journey, and every contribution, no matter how small, can make a difference. Whether you're helping individuals, animals, or the environment, your efforts contribute to building a better world.

Social support networks play a crucial role in maintaining physical, emotional, and psychological well-being for individuals across various aspects of life. These networks consist of family, friends, peers, colleagues, and community members who provide assistance, empathy, companionship, and resources. The importance of social support networks can be understood from several perspectives:

1. Emotional Well-being: Social support networks offer a platform for individuals to share their feelings, concerns, and experiences. Having someone to talk to can alleviate feelings of loneliness, anxiety, and depression. Emotional support from loved ones can provide comfort during challenging times, reducing the negative impact of stressors.

2. Stress Reduction: Strong social support networks help individuals cope with stress more effectively. People who have access to emotional and practical support are better equipped to handle life's challenges and recover from adversity.

3. Mental Health: Regular interactions and connections with others can contribute to improved mental health outcomes. Individuals with a strong social support system are less likely to experience severe mental health issues and are more likely to seek help when needed.

4. Physical Health: Social support has been linked to

improved physical health outcomes. Having people who encourage healthy behaviors, such as exercising or eating well, can positively impact an individual's overall health.

5. Sense of Belonging: Social support networks provide a sense of belonging and acceptance. This sense of community helps individuals feel valued and understood, reducing feelings of isolation and fostering a positive self-image.

6. Coping with Life Transitions: During significant life transitions like relocating to a new place, beginning a new job, or going through a loss, social support networks provide direction and stability. They help individuals navigate unfamiliar situations and adapt to changes.

7. Problem Solving and Advice: Social support networks provide access to diverse perspectives and experiences. This can be invaluable when seeking advice, brainstorming solutions, or making important decisions.

8. Building Resilience: Having a strong social support system contributes to an individual's resilience. Supportive relationships provide a buffer against negative experiences, helping people bounce back from setbacks.

9. Positive Behaviors: Individuals in supportive networks often influence each other to engage in positive behaviors. This can include adopting

healthier habits, pursuing personal goals, and maintaining a positive outlook on life.

10. Longevity: Studies suggest that individuals with robust social support networks tend to live longer and experience a higher quality of life. This could be due to the combination of emotional, mental, and physical benefits provided by such networks

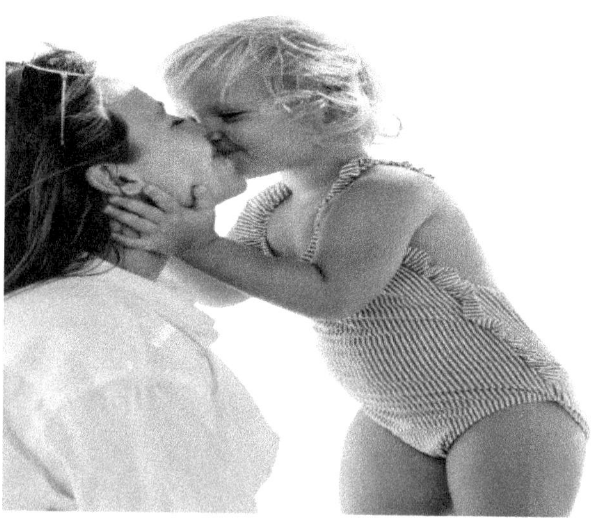

CHAPTER FIVE

SPIRITUAL WELLNESS

Spiritual wellness is one of the dimensions of overall well-being, alongside physical, emotional, mental, and social wellness. It refers to the pursuit of meaning and purpose in life as well as a feeling of being connected to something bigger than oneself. While spiritual wellness often has roots in religious or philosophical beliefs, it can also be experienced in a more secular and individualized manner.

Key aspects of spiritual wellness include

1. Meaning and Purpose: Individuals with high spiritual wellness often feel a sense of purpose and meaning in their lives. They have a clear understanding of their values and how those values contribute to their overall life goals.

2. Connection: Spiritual wellness involves feeling connected to something beyond oneself. This could be a higher power, nature, the universe, or a sense of interconnectedness with all living beings.

3. Inner Peace: A strong spiritual foundation can provide a sense of inner peace and tranquility. People with high spiritual wellness often experience a greater ability to cope with stress and challenges.

4. Self-Reflection: Spiritual wellness encourages self-

reflection and introspection. It involves exploring questions about the nature of existence, morality, and the deeper aspects of life.

5. Practices and Rituals: Many people engage in spiritual practices and rituals that align with their beliefs. These could include meditation, prayer, and mindfulness, yoga, attending religious services, or participating in other forms of contemplative activities.

6. Compassion and Empathy: Spiritual wellness often leads to a greater sense of compassion and empathy for others. It promotes a deeper understanding of the human experience and encourages acts of kindness and service.

7. Resilience: Having a strong spiritual foundation can contribute to emotional resilience. It provides a source of support and comfort during challenging times and can help individuals bounce back from adversity.

8. Balance: Achieving spiritual wellness involves finding a balance between the demands of daily life and the need for introspection and connection. It's about integrating these aspects into one's overall well-being.

It's important to note that spiritual wellness is a deeply personal and individualized experience. What brings a sense of meaning, connection, and purpose to one person may differ from another. Some individuals find spiritual wellness through organized religion, while others find it through nature, philosophy, or personal exploration.

Cultivating spiritual wellness often requires ongoing self-discovery, open-mindedness, and willingness to EXPLORE DIFFERENT BELIEFS AND PRACTICES. It's a lifelong journey that can contribute significantly to a person's overall sense of well-being and fulfillment.

Exploring beliefs and values can be a deeply introspective and thought-provoking endeavor. Let's break down these concepts:

Beliefs:

Beliefs are the convictions or opinions that individuals hold to be true. They can be influenced by personal experiences, upbringing, culture, religion, education, and more. Beliefs can encompass a wide range of topics, including factual information, philosophical concepts, moral judgments, and even assumptions about the world. Some beliefs are conscious and well-formed, while others might be subconscious or implicit. It's important to note that beliefs can vary widely among individuals, and people may hold contradictory beliefs.

Values:

Values are guiding principles or ideals that influence

how individuals perceive and interact with the world around them. They provide a framework for decision-making, behavior, and prioritization. Values can be intrinsic (core values that are deeply ingrained) or extrinsic (values that are influenced by external factors like society or peers). They often reflect what someone considers important, meaningful, and worthwhile in life. Examples of values include honesty, compassion, freedom, justice, family, and personal growth.

Exploring Beliefs:

1. Self-Reflection: Take time to reflect on your own beliefs. What do you believe about life, the universe, morality, and other significant topics? Ask yourself where these beliefs came from and why you hold them.

2. Questioning: Challenge your beliefs by asking critical questions. Are your beliefs based on evidence and reason, or are they influenced by biases or assumptions? Consider whether your beliefs have evolved over time and why.

3. Open-Mindedness: Be open to different perspectives. Have discussions with folks who have different worldviews. This can help you understand alternative viewpoints and potentially refine your own beliefs.

4. Research: If your beliefs are related to factual matters, engage in research to ensure your

understanding is accurate and up-to-date Information and knowledge can evolve throughout time.

Knowledge and information can change over time.

Exploring Values:

1. Identify Core Values: Make a list of values that resonate with you. Consider what values are most important in your life. This can serve as a foundation for your decision-making process.

2. Reflect on Life Choices: Think about significant decisions you've made and analyze how your values influenced those decisions. Did your values align with your choices, or did you compromise them?

3. Prioritization: Sometimes, values might conflict, and you might need to prioritize one over the other. Consider how you prioritize your values in different situations and what factors influence those choices.

4. Personal Growth: Values can evolve as you gain new experiences and insights. Continuously reflect on whether your values still hold true or if they need adjustments.

5. Consistency: Strive for consistency between your values and actions. Living in alignment with your values can lead to a more fulfilling and authentic life.

Remember that beliefs and values are deeply personal, and there's no one-size-fits-all approach to exploring them. It's an ongoing process that requires self-awareness, introspection, and a willingness to adapt as you learn and grow.

Self-reflection and personal growth are interconnected processes that involve introspection, awareness, and intentional development. They are essential aspects of human development that allow individuals to better understand themselves, their values, beliefs, behaviors, and emotions. Knowledge and information can develop through time.

Self-Reflection:

Self-reflection is the practice of examining your thoughts, feelings, and experiences in a thoughtful and introspective manner. It involves taking the time to pause, analyze, and gain insights into your actions, decisions, and reactions. Self-reflection can be done through various methods, such as journaling, meditation, mindfulness, or conversations with trusted friends or mentors.

Key aspects of self-reflection include:

1. Awareness: It starts with becoming aware of your thoughts, emotions, and behaviors in different situations. This awareness allows you to identify patterns, triggers, and areas of your life that might need attention.

2. Questioning: Ask yourself probing questions to explore your motivations, fears, aspirations, and values. This helps you delve deeper into your thoughts and feelings to uncover underlying reasons for your actions.

3. Learning from Mistakes: Reflecting on your mistakes and failures can provide valuable lessons. Understanding what went wrong and why can help you make better decisions in the future.

4. Growth Mindset: Embracing a growth mindset involves believing in your capacity to change and improve. Self-reflection supports this mindset by helping you identify areas for growth and development.

Personal Growth:

Personal growth is the intentional process of developing and enhancing various aspects of your life to become a better version of yourself. It encompasses emotional, intellectual, physical, and spiritual dimensions. Personal growth is not about comparing yourself to others; instead, it's about measuring your progress against your own potential.

Key elements of personal growth include:

1. Setting Goals: Establishing clear and achievable goals helps you have a direction for your growth journey. These goals can relate to different areas of your life, such as career, relationships, health, and

skills.

2. Continuous Learning: Engaging in lifelong learning fosters personal growth. This could involve acquiring new skills, seeking new experiences, reading books, attending workshops, or pursuing formal education.

3. Stepping Out of Comfort Zones: Growth often occurs outside of your comfort zone. Taking calculated risks and facing challenges can lead to personal development and increased self-confidence.

4. Cultivating Positive Habits: Developing healthy habits, such as regular exercise, balanced nutrition, effective time management, and consistent self-care, contributes to your overall growth and well-being.

5. Emotional Intelligence: Enhancing your emotional intelligence enables better understanding and management of your emotions and relationships. This skill is crucial for personal growth and effective communication. Spiritual fulfillment can be pursued through a variety of paths, and the approach that resonates with one person might differ from another. Here are some different paths to spiritual fulfillment:

1. Religious Practice: Many people find spiritual fulfillment through organized religions. Following rituals, engaging in prayer, participating in community activities, and studying sacred texts can provide a sense of connection to something greater than oneself.

2. Meditation and Mindfulness: Meditation and mindfulness practices focus on being present in the moment, calming the mind, and connecting with inner peace. These practices can lead to self-awareness, reduced stress, and a deeper sense of spirituality.

3. Nature Connection: Spending time in nature can help individuals feel connected to the natural world and find a sense of wonder and awe. This can lead to feelings of interconnectedness and a deeper appreciation for the universe.

4. Service and Compassion: Engaging in acts of service and showing compassion towards others can provide a sense of purpose and fulfillment. Helping others and making a positive impact on the world can be deeply spiritually rewarding.

5. Creative Expression: Pursuing creative endeavors like art, music, writing, or dance can be a way to tap into one's inner self and express emotions and thoughts that might be difficult to convey through words alone.

6. Yoga and Movement: Yoga is a physical, mental, and spiritual practice that combines movement, breath control, and meditation. It aims to harmonize the body and mind, leading to a greater sense of balance and spiritual connection.

7. Philosophical Inquiry: Engaging in philosophical and existential questions can lead to a deeper

understanding of oneself, one's purpose, and the nature of reality. Exploring different philosophies and belief systems can be a path to spiritual growth.

8. Study and Learning: Delving into spiritual and philosophical literature, as well as studying the teachings of various spiritual leaders, can provide intellectual and spiritual growth.

9. Simplicity and Minimalism: Embracing a simple and minimalist lifestyle can help individuals detach from material possessions and focus on what truly matters, fostering a deeper sense of contentment and spiritual connection.

10. Personal Growth and Self-Discovery: Engaging in practices that promote self-awareness, emotional healing, and personal growth can lead to a more profound understanding of oneself and one's spiritual journey.

11. Contemplative Practices: Practices that involve deep contemplation, introspection, and self-inquiry can help individuals connect with their inner wisdom and experience spiritual insights.

12. Transcendent Experiences: Some people have spiritual experiences through moments of awe, near-death experiences, or other transcendent events that lead to a profound shift in their understanding of reality and spirituality.

The mind-body-spirit connection

refers to the interrelationship between our mental, physical, and spiritual well-being. It is a holistic concept that suggests these three aspects of our being are interconnected and influence each other's health and functioning. Here's a breakdown of each component:

1. Mind: The mind encompasses our thoughts, emotions, beliefs, and cognitive processes. It plays a crucial role in shaping our perceptions, behaviors, and overall mental health. Positive thoughts and emotional well-being can have beneficial effects on physical health and spiritual growth.

2. Body: The body represents our physical form and includes our organs, systems, and physiological processes. Physical health directly affects mental and emotional well-being. For instance, regular exercise, a balanced diet, sufficient sleep, and stress management can contribute to improved mental health and spiritual growth.

3. Spirit: The spirit or soul is often associated with a person's inner essence or consciousness. It involves aspects of purpose, meaning, values, and the search for deeper understanding. Spiritual well-being can positively impact mental and physical health by providing a sense of purpose, hope, and resilience

The concept of the mind-body-spirit connection suggests that imbalances or disruptions in one aspect can affect the others. For instance:

- Mental distress, such as chronic stress or anxiety, can lead to physical symptoms like headaches, digestive issues, or weakened immune function.

- Physical ailments, such as chronic pain or illness, can contribute to emotional challenges like depression or frustration.

- Spiritual disconnect or lack of purpose can result in feelings of emptiness, lack of motivation, and contribute to mental health issues.

Recognizing and nurturing the mind-body-spirit connection can lead to a more holistic approach to well-being. Practices such as meditation, mindfulness, yoga, prayer, journaling, and engaging in hobbies that bring joy can help strengthen this connection. Integrating these practices can promote overall health and help individuals achieve greater balance and harmony in their lives. It's important to note that different cultures and belief systems may interpret and approach the mind-body-spirit connection in various ways.

Practices of inner peace can greatly enhance your mental, emotional, and spiritual well-being. Cultivating inner peace involves adopting various habits and techniques that help you manage stress, reduce anxiety, and achieve a sense of calm and contentment. Here are some methods you might want to use:

1. Meditation: Regular meditation practice can help

calm your mind, increase self-awareness, and reduce stress. Mindfulness meditation, loving-kindness meditation, and transcendental meditation are a few popular types.

2. Deep Breathing: Practicing deep and slow breathing can activate your body's relaxation response and help you stay grounded. Techniques like diaphragmatic breathing or the 4-7-8 breathing pattern can be effective.

3. Yoga: Yoga combines physical postures, breathing exercises, and meditation. It promotes flexibility, balance, and relaxation while also fostering a connection between your mind and body.

4. Mindfulness: Being present in the moment and fully engaged in whatever you're doing can help you appreciate the simple joys of life and reduce overthinking.

5. Gratitude: Practicing gratitude involves focusing on the positive aspects of your life and acknowledging the things you are thankful for. Your attention may be drawn from the negative in this way.

6. Journaling: Writing down your thoughts, feelings, and experiences can provide a healthy outlet for emotions and help you gain insights into your inner world.

7. Nature Connection: Spending time in nature can have a calming and grounding effect on your mind.

Take walks, sit outdoors, or engage in activities like hiking to connect with the natural world.

8. Limiting Media Consumption: Reduce exposure to negative news and excessive social media to prevent unnecessary stress and anxiety.

9. Physical Exercise: Regular physical activity not only benefits your physical health but also releases endorphins that improve your mood and overall sense of well-being.

10. Healthy Lifestyle: Prioritize proper sleep, maintain a balanced diet, and avoid excessive caffeine or alcohol, as they can impact your emotional equilibrium.

11. Creativity and Hobbies: Engaging in creative pursuits or hobbies you enjoy can provide a sense of accomplishment and joy, promoting inner peace.

12. Spend Time with Loved Ones: Connecting with family and friends who uplift and support you can contribute to your emotional well-being.

13. Practice Forgiveness: Let go of grudges and practice forgiveness, both for yourself and others. Holding onto resentment can hinder inner peace.

14. Volunteer Work: Contributing to your community or helping others in need can foster a sense of purpose and fulfillment.

15. Mindful Eating: Pay attention to your meals and

savor the flavors. Eating mindfully can help you develop a healthier relationship with food and increase your overall mindfulness.

Remember that achieving inner peace is a journey and may require patience and consistency. It's also important to find practices that resonate with you personally and integrate them into your daily routine. Over time, these practices can help you cultivate a deeper sense of calm, balance, and contentment in your life.

Meditation and contemplation are both practices that involve focused attention and mental exercises, but they have distinct characteristics and purposes. Let's explore each of them:

Meditation:

Meditation is a mental practice that aims to achieve a state of deep relaxation and heightened awareness. It involves focusing the mind and eliminating distractions to promote mental clarity, emotional calmness, and overall well-being. There are many different types of meditation, each with unique practices and objectives. Some common types of meditation include:

1. Mindfulness Meditation: This involves paying non-judgmental attention to the present moment, including your thoughts, sensations, and emotions.

2. Transcendental Meditation: A technique where you

repeat a specific mantra to achieve a state of deep relaxation and reduced mental activity.

3. Loving-kindness Meditation: This practice focuses on developing feelings of compassion and empathy towards oneself and others.

4. Breath Awareness Meditation: The focus is on observing and regulating the breath to bring about relaxation and mental clarity.

5. Guided Meditation: In this form, a guide leads you through a mental journey or visualization, often with the aim of achieving specific goals like stress reduction or personal growth.

Contemplation:

Contemplation, on the other hand, involves deep thinking, reflection, and intellectual exploration of a particular subject or idea. It is often more active and cognitive compared to some forms of meditation. Contemplation encourages critical thinking and analyzing the complexities of a topic. It might involve pondering philosophical questions, exploring ethical dilemmas, or considering the deeper meaning of life.

Contemplation can be more structured and guided by asking questions, reading texts, or engaging in discussions. It's a practice that seeks understanding and insight by delving into the layers of a subject and examining it from multiple angles.

Key Differences:

1. Focus: Meditation involves calming the mind and reducing mental activity, often through techniques like breath awareness. Contemplation involves active thinking and reflecting on a specific topic.

2. Goal: The goal of meditation is often relaxation, heightened awareness, and emotional balance. Contemplation seeks to deepen understanding and gain insights into a subject.

3. Approach: Meditation often involves techniques to quiet the mind and let go of thoughts. Contemplation encourages the exploration and analysis of thoughts and ideas.

4. State of Mind: Meditation often aims to achieve a state of mental stillness and present-moment awareness. Contemplation engages the mind in an active process of thinking and reasoning.

Yoga and Tai Chi are both ancient practices that offer numerous physical, mental, and spiritual benefits. They are often associated with improving flexibility, balance, relaxation, and overall well-being. However, they have different origins, philosophies, and techniques.

Yoga:

Yoga originated in ancient India and has a rich history spanning thousands of years. It encompasses a wide range of practices that aim to unify the mind, body, and spirit. Yoga comes in a variety of forms, each with its own emphasis and methodology. Some popular styles include Hatha, Vinyasa, Ashtanga, Iyengar, and Kundalini yoga.

Yoga typically involves a combination of physical postures (asanas), breathing exercises (pranayama), meditation, and ethical principles for living (yamas and niyamas). It emphasizes the connection between breath and movement, helping practitioners become more aware of their bodies and minds. Yoga is known for its holistic approach to health and well-being, promoting flexibility, strength, relaxation, stress reduction, and inner peace.

Tai Chi:

Tai Chi, also known as Tai Chi Chuan, originated in China and is a martial art that has evolved into a graceful form of exercise and meditation. It is characterized by slow, flowing movements and deep, relaxed breathing. Tai Chi is often practiced as a series of choreographed movements known as forms, which are performed in a continuous, mindful manner.

Tai Chi is based on the principles of balance, harmony, and the circulation of vital energy (Qi or Chi) throughout the body. It aims to improve the flow of energy, enhance physical and mental relaxation, and develop body awareness and coordination. Tai Chi is particularly known for its benefits in promoting balance, reducing stress, improving posture, and enhancing flexibility and joint mobility.

Both yoga and Tai Chi can be adapted to various fitness levels and age groups. They are practiced by people seeking physical exercise, stress relief, improved mental clarity, and spiritual growth. While yoga often involves holding poses and stretching, Tai Chi focuses on continuous, fluid movements. The decision between the two is based on personal preferences, objectives, and health factors.

Nature connection and eco-spirituality are concepts that revolve around the relationship between humans and the natural world, and how this connection can lead to a deeper sense of spirituality and interconnectedness with all life forms and the environment. Let's delve deeper into each of these ideas:

1. Nature Connection:

Nature connection refers to the idea of fostering a strong and meaningful relationship with the natural world. This involves spending time in nature, observing its beauty, understanding its cycles, and recognizing the interdependence of all living beings. It's about recognizing our place within the larger ecosystem and acknowledging the benefits and inspiration that nature provides to us.

Connecting with nature has been associated with numerous physical, mental, and emotional benefits, including reduced stress, improved mood, enhanced creativity, and a greater sense of well-being. Practices like hiking, camping, gardening, and mindfulness in natural settings can help individuals develop a stronger bond with the environment.

2. Eco-Spirituality:

Eco-spirituality, sometimes referred to as ecological spirituality or Earth-based spirituality, is a belief system that incorporates ecological awareness and reverence for the natural world into one's spiritual framework. It recognizes the interconnectedness of all life forms and views nature as sacred and worthy of protection and care.

Eco-spirituality often emphasizes the idea that the Earth is not just a resource for human use, but a living entity with its own intrinsic value. It encourages practices that honor and respect the environment, such as sustainable living, ethical consumption, and environmental activism. Many eco-spiritual traditions draw inspiration from indigenous wisdom, ancient religious beliefs, and philosophical perspectives that celebrate the harmony between humans and nature.

Some common themes within eco-spirituality include:

- Deep Ecology: This philosophical perspective views all life as interconnected and stresses the importance of addressing ecological issues at their root causes. It encourages a shift in values from human-centered to Earth-centered.

- Gaia Hypothesis: Proposed by James Lovelock, this hypothesis suggests that the Earth functions as a self-regulating organism, with living and non-living components working together to maintain a stable environment.

- Animism: This belief holds that all elements of the natural world possess a spiritual essence or consciousness. It's a common perspective in many indigenous cultures.

- Transcendence through Nature: Some people find spiritual enlightenment and connection with the divine through their experiences in nature, seeing it as a source of awe and wonder that can lead to deeper understanding and insight.

Overall, nature connection and eco-spirituality offer pathways for individuals to cultivate a more profound relationship with the Earth and a sense of purpose that extends beyond human concerns. These concepts can provide a framework for addressing environmental challenges and promoting a more sustainable and harmonious world

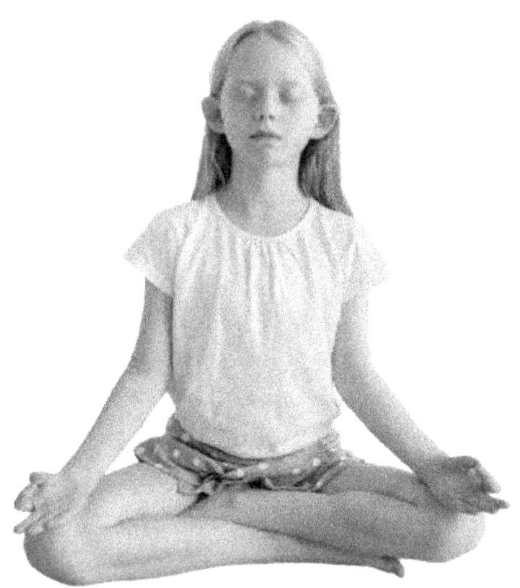

CHAPTER SIX

LIVING A LIFE OF WELLNESS AND VITALITY

Living a life of wellness and vitality involves making conscious choices and adopting habits that promote your physical, mental, and emotional well-being. Consider the following important guidelines and practices:

1. Balanced Nutrition: Eat a well-rounded diet rich in fruits, vegetables, whole grains, lean proteins, and healthy fats. Stay hydrated and avoids excessive consumption of processed foods, sugary snacks, and beverages.

2. Regular Exercise: Engage in regular physical activity that suits your fitness level and preferences. Exercises like yoga and swimming can be included in this, along with cardio, strength, and flexibility drills.

3. Adequate Sleep: Prioritize quality sleep by establishing a consistent sleep schedule, creating a calming bedtime routine, and maintaining a comfortable sleep environment. Adults typically require 7-9 hours of sleep per night.

4. Stress Management: Practice stress-reduction techniques such as meditation, deep breathing, mindfulness, and relaxation exercises. Engaging in

hobbies, spending time in nature, and socializing can also help alleviate stress.

5. Positive Relationships: Cultivate meaningful connections with friends, family, and loved ones. Strong social bonds contribute to emotional well-being and provide a support system during challenging times.

6. Mental and Emotional Health: Prioritize self-care and mental health by seeking professional help when needed, practicing self-compassion, setting healthy boundaries, and engaging in activities that bring you joy.

7. Mindful Living: Practice mindfulness by being present in the moment and paying attention to your thoughts, feelings, and surroundings. This can enhance your overall awareness and reduce feelings of anxiety or overwhelm.

8. Hygiene and Self-Care: Maintain good personal hygiene, including regular grooming, skincare, and dental care. Take part in relaxing and esteem-boosting self-care exercises.

9. Continuous Learning: Keep your mind active by engaging in lifelong learning. This could involve reading, taking up new hobbies, attending classes or workshops, and staying curious about the world around you.

10. Limiting Harmful Habits: Reduce or eliminate habits that can negatively impact your well-being, such as smoking, excessive alcohol consumption, and recreational drug use.

11. Gratitude Practice: Cultivate an attitude of gratitude by regularly acknowledging and appreciating the positive aspects of your life. This can improve your overall outlook and satisfaction.

12. Setting Goals: Set achievable goals for various areas of your life, such as health, career, relationships, and personal growth. Working toward these goals can give you a sense of purpose and accomplishment.

Remember that wellness and vitality are ongoing pursuits, and everyone's journey is unique. It's important to find a balance that works for you and to make gradual, sustainable changes. Consulting with healthcare professionals, such as doctors, nutritionists, and mental health therapists, can provide personalized guidance based on your individual needs and circumstances.

Celebrating achievements is a wonderful way to acknowledge and recognize the hard work, dedication, and success that someone has accomplished. Whether it's a personal achievement or a milestone reached within a professional or academic context, celebrating helps boost morale, motivation, and overall well-being. Here are some ideas on how to celebrate achievements:

1. Throw a Party or Gathering: Organize a gathering with friends, family, or colleagues to celebrate the achievement. It could be a casual get-together, a themed party, or a formal event, depending on the significance of the achievement.

2. Personal Treat: Treat yourself or the achiever to something special, like a spa day, a favorite meal at a nice restaurant, or a weekend getaway.

3. Gifts: Consider giving a thoughtful gift that reflects the achievement. This could be something related to the accomplishment, a personalized item, or something the person has been wanting for a while.

4. Recognition: Publicly recognize the achievement. This could be through a social media post, a company-wide announcement, or an article in a newsletter.

5. Certificates and Awards: Create a certificate or award that commemorates the achievement. This is especially meaningful for academic or professional accomplishments.

6. Charitable Donation: Make a donation to a charity or cause that's important to the achiever. This can be a meaningful way to give back while celebrating success.

7. Customized Celebration: Tailor the celebration to the individual's interests. If they love sports, consider organizing a sports-related event. If they enjoy the

arts, plan a cultural outing.

8. Time with Loved Ones: Sometimes, simply spending quality time with family and friends can be the best way to celebrate. Engage in activities you all enjoy together.

9. Words of Encouragement: Write a heartfelt letter or card expressing your pride and admiration for the person's accomplishment. Speaking kind words can leave a lasting impression.

10. Reflection: Take time to reflect on the journey that led to the achievement. Share stories, challenges overcome, and lessons learned.

11. Professional Development: For career-related achievements, investing in further professional development or education could be a meaningful way to celebrate.

12. Creative Expression: Create something artistic or crafty to commemorate the achievement. This could be a scrapbook, a painting, a song, or any form of creative expression.

Remember, the key is to make the celebration meaningful and tailored to the individual's preferences and the nature of the achievement. It's a time to honor their hard work and dedication, and to inspire them to continue reaching for even greater heights in the future.

Commitment to ongoing self-care is a vital aspect of maintaining one's physical, mental, and emotional well-being. It involves consistently engaging in activities and practices that promote health, reduce stress, and enhance overall quality of life. Here are some key principles and tips for fostering a strong commitment to ongoing self-care:

1. Prioritize Self-Care: Recognize that self-care is not a selfish indulgence but a necessary practice to maintain your overall health and resilience. Put it first in your daily or weekly schedule.

2. Create a Routine: Establish a regular schedule for self-care activities. Consistency is the key to reaping the long-term benefits of self-care.

3. Holistic Approach: Self-care should address various aspects of your well-being, including physical, emotional, mental, and spiritual health. Find a balance between these dimensions.

4. Know Yourself: Understand your personal needs, preferences, and limits. What works for someone else might not work for you, so tailor your self-care practices accordingly.

5. Set Boundaries: Learn to say no to commitments or activities that drain your energy or cause unnecessary stress. Maintaining your wellbeing requires establishing sound limits.

6. Physical Health: Engage in regular exercise, maintain a balanced diet, get sufficient sleep, and attend regular medical check-ups. These fundamental practices contribute to your overall vitality.

7. Mental and Emotional Health: Practice mindfulness, meditation, deep breathing, or journaling to manage stress and enhance emotional well-being. Engage in activities that bring you joy and relaxation.

8. Social Connections: Foster positive relationships with friends, family, and loved ones. Spend quality time with people who uplift and support you.

9. Hobbies and Interests: Make time for activities you enjoy, whether it's reading, painting, playing a musical instrument, gardening, or any other hobby that brings you happiness.

10. Learn to Say Yes to Yourself: Just as you say yes to commitments and responsibilities, remember to say yes to your own needs. Make time for yourself without feeling guilty.

11. Adapt and Evolve: Life circumstances change, so be prepared to adjust your self-care routine as needed. Flexibility is important in maintaining your commitment to self-care.

12. Avoid Overextending: While it's important to challenge yourself, be cautious not to overextend yourself to the point of burnout. Recognize your

limits and give yourself permission to rest.

13. Self-Compassion: Treat yourself with kindness and understanding. If you miss a self-care activity or have a setback, don't be too hard on yourself. Self-compassion is a key component of ongoing self-care.

14. Seek Professional Help: If you're struggling with your commitment to self-care or facing persistent challenges, consider seeking guidance from a therapist, counselor, or healthcare professional.

Self-care is a journey, not a destination. It requires ongoing effort and dedication to maintain a healthy and balanced life. By consistently investing in your well-being, you'll be better equipped to navigate life's challenges and enjoy its reward

ABOUT THE AUTHOR

Author Name: Kelvin Williams

Kelvin Williams is a renowned expert in the field of holistic health and wellness. With a background in both conventional medicine and alternative healing practices, he has dedicated his life to helping people achieve optimal well-being and vitality. Kelvin's journey began with a degree in traditional medicine, but his curiosity led him to explore various holistic approaches from around the world.